Love Unlimited

The Joys and Challenges of Open Relationships

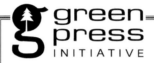

Love Unlimited

The Joys and Challenges of Open Relationships

Leonie Linssen and Stephan Wik

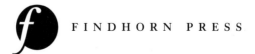

FINDHORN PRESS

©Leonie Linssen and Stephan Wik, 2010

The right of Leonie Linssen and Stephan Wik to be
identified as the authors of this work has been asserted by them
in accordance with the Copyright, Designs and Patents Act 1998.

Published in 2010 by Findhorn Press, Scotland

ISBN 978-1-84409-183-6

A CIP record for this title is available from the British Library.

Edited by Victoria Stahl
Cover design by Aude Ferrière
Interior design by Damian Keenan
Printed and bound in the USA

1 2 3 4 5 6 7 8 9 17 16 15 14 13 12 11 10

Published by
Findhorn Press
117-121 High Street,
Forres IV36 1AB,
Scotland, UK

t +44 (0)1309 690582
f +44 (0)131 777 2711
e info@findhornpress.com
www.findhornpress.com

Contents

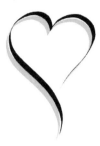

Leonie's
Introduction

In 2005, I started my own coaching practice, *Verander je Wereld* (*Change Your World*) with a mission to teach people how to live a life of authenticity, and thereby create successful relationships based on passion and power. At about the same time, I attended a seminar given by Pim van Lommel, who has conducted scientific research on near-death experiences. The stories from people who have had near-death experiences touched me deeply, as they had all experienced a world of complete love and total compassion for others — without judgements. The experiences they described totally matched the underlying foundations of my counseling work and my personal life.

I had recently experienced how healing it can be to form a relationship with someone from the space of complete acceptance. My life partner, soon after meeting me for the first time, had challenged me to accept myself completely. This meant accepting all the facets of my being, even in the areas of relationships and sexuality. So the seminar really brought both aspects together — professional and personal — and I realized, *yes*, this is what I have to offer the world. The talk by Pim was, for me, a clear confirmation that I had made the right choice when I decided to start working as a relationship coach for people in complex intimate relationships. This was really important for me, as I'm a pioneer in this area of coaching in the Netherlands.

I grew up in a small Dutch village with an upbringing based on monogamy, strict rules and the Catholic faith. My childhood concepts of love and relationships were rather romantic, and bore no relation to who I actually was. For instance, at the age of fourteen I already knew that I was not only attracted to boys, but also to girls. That definitely didn't fit into my storybook picture! When I was nineteen I found myself in love with three people at the same time, and this was completely at odds with the "correct" way to behave. Unfortunately, I didn't know anyone else who admitted to these kinds of feelings, and I couldn't find a way to come to terms with who I was. For years and years I suppressed my desires until suddenly, at the age of forty, they surfaced again with a vengeance and I was forced to take a good, hard look at myself.

Societal pressure to conform is huge. Someone who wants to live a life based on true personal authenticity first has to have the courage to be who he or she really is. For many of us, this is an in-depth process that first involves discovering how to come into contact with our own inner source of truth, our core being. After honestly looking inside, we start to become conscious of how we have been taught to behave, our inherited and often indiscriminate beliefs, our mental and emotional blocks, the values and norms we hold to be true, and of course the role of the ego.

My subsequent personal journey of discovery in the area of relationships and sexuality was a powerful, and at the same time difficult, transformation process. It made such a strong impression on me that I decided I would like to share my experiences and, if possible, be of service to others grappling with the same issues. I imagined how wonderful it would be to help other people. In particular, I was interested in helping people discover exactly what works for them, as I saw what a difference it makes to be in a relationship form that suits our individual needs. So, I went back to university, earned a degree in counseling, and after many, many workshops and seminars, my practice was born.

Since then, I've coached hundreds of people about their relationships. Most of these people are struggling with the fact that they have romantic feelings and/or are sexually attracted to someone other than their partners. They are searching for ways to accept and deal with their feelings in a society where monogamy and heterosexuality are still, for a very large part, considered the norm. Many of my clients judge themselves harshly for what they are feeling or for what they have done, while others are struggling with their partners' needs for more freedom within the context of their intimate relationships.

After a while, I clearly realized that something needed to be done to break through the taboo around alternative forms of intimate relationships, and at the very least, I wanted to take part in making it possible to talk freely and honestly about open relationships and polyamory. Until I met the Swedish/American author Stephan Wik, I hadn't worked out how to do this. However, he'd read about my work on a Dutch web site and was very enthusiastic about it. After many extensive and intensive talks it became clear to both of us: we were going to write a (this!) book together. Or as Stephan put it: "This book needs to be written and I guess we're the ones who need to do it!"

Love Unlimited is a compilation of twelve case studies. The people portrayed are struggling with challenges that have arisen as a result of romantic or sexual feelings they are experiencing, which are outside monogamous models. The stories are based on the experiences of a large number of real people. We've created the stories out of material that has emerged from hundreds of counseling sessions, discussions with experts in the field of love and relationships, publications and specialized Internet forums, talks with friends and our own experiences.

The stories in *Love Unlimited* follow people from the point that they reach an impasse, then through their coaching processes until they're ready to carry on under their own steam. We describe the coaching and the periods between the coaching sessions, and provide a great deal of background information on the topics covered in each story. In addition, Stephan adds another dimension to *Love Unlimited*. He has extensive knowledge of other ancient cultural practices, such as Taoist sacred sexuality, where sexual energy is used as a source of energy for physical healing and spiritual development. His contributions encourage the reader to consider the fact that there are other ways of viewing both relationships and sexuality, and to realize that our Western paradigm is not the only one. Each chapter ends with tips and reflections on the topics covered. These gently challenge the reader to incorporate the ideas and tools into their own lives.

Recently, I took part in a meditation weekend (Satsang) where I experienced an expansion of my consciousness, which allowed me to view the world "from the other side." It became clear to me that, ultimately, we are all connected to each other through love. Love is all that is left when the judgements that we have about ourselves and others are released. It has been the most wonderful experience in my life, and it has made it absolutely clear to me why *Love Unlimited* needed to be written. As people on this planet, we all have our negative thoughts that restrict us or hold us back from what we want to achieve: a happy life with room for individuality, passion and sustainable intimate relationships. The ideas addressed in *Love Unlimited* can help us move in this direction, as they offer insight into a challenging new world where there is room for more love, and more personal growth.

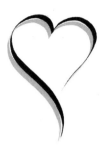

Stephan's
Introduction

The softest things in the world
overcome the hardest things in the world.
—*LAO TZU*

This book started when I was doing research for what I thought was going to be my own next book. My previous book, written with my wife Mieke, was about Taoist Sacred Sexuality and describes how we discovered the ancient Taoist healing tradition of working consciously with sexual energy. Shortly after that book was published, our friends encouraged us to offer workshops to others who might be interested in this information. So we took a plunge into the unknown and spent eighteen months giving workshops and meeting people interested in learning more about working consciously with sexual energy.

It didn't take long before I started to see an interesting pattern emerging from the participants, usually couples, that we met during this time. Our initial contact with couples was usually based on their interest in our book and specifically the topic of working consciously with sexual energy. However we soon discovered that the real issue that people wanted to talk about was not so much about how to work with sexual energy, but how to talk to each other. They wanted to learn how to communicate openly and honestly about intimate issues, without fear or shame and without guilt or blame. We were amazed at how many people said that we were the first people they had ever been able to talk to about these issues. We were quite touched by people's openness and trust in us, especially as we are not counsellors or coaches. It seemed that the fact that we were prepared to speak openly and honestly about our own experiences made it possible for other people to open up and speak to us and to each other.

And that was how I found Leonie. I was researching tools for clear communication on the Internet and I saw an article from a coach and counsellor who wrote in a wonderfully clear and succinct fashion. I was intrigued and decided to contact her. We met up a few months later and decided to collaborate on this book.

Why, with my background in Taoist Energy work, would I want to write a book with someone who specializes in non-traditional relationships and polyamory? What's the connection? In a word, "softening." In Taoist Healing work there is a common thread or understanding that states that our lives are dependent on a healthy flow of Life Energy through our entire body, mind and spirit system. Rigidity, whether physical, emotional or intellectual, can create obstructions to this life-enhancing flow of life energy. Given enough obstructions and rigidity, the life energy can be hindered in its flow with negative effects on our health and wellbeing.

As I talked to Leonie, I discovered that her interpretations, and the healthy-relationship tools she works with, are based on the very same principle. If you have rigidity and stiffness in your relationship, the health of the relationship will suffer and, sooner or later, it will probably come to an end. So learning how to be flexible, open, relaxed and free within a relationship is really the key to not only its survival but also its growth and well-being. Leonie helps people, singles and those in relationships, learn to relax, step back, observe and then take conscious steps to create a healthy energy flow between all concerned. The tools and techniques that have been developed to help people deal with issues that arise in polyamorous and open relationships are valuable to all of us no matter what forms our personal relationships take.

When I came across Leonie I also heard about the term "polyamory" for the first time and started to read discussions from, and ultimately meet, many people who consider themselves "polyamorous." I am struck by the fact that so many of the people who are exploring this area are so level-headed and clear about how to develop new ways of dealing with the emotional ups and downs of relationships. It is particularly fascinating to realize that many of the people I have met and spoken with at length are actually in monogamous relationships and are simply exploring the boundaries of their relationships. They aren't actively engaged with people outside their relationships and many of them never have been. However, the experience of communicating honestly about the possibility of opening up their relationships has brought new and higher levels of honesty, communication and sharing into their lives. I see this over and over again.

One of the key skills these people have learned is something the Taoists also speak of — to recognize, acknowledge, accept and then release strong emotions. For example, they have learned to accept that, yes, they will probably be a bit jealous when their partners talk about someone else and/or spend time with them. But they don't have to judge themselves or try to suppress their feelings, they simply accept them and learn to take care of themselves when this happens by, for instance, doing something they like. After a while they notice that their responses are not as strong and that the emotional storms are not nearly as severe. They begin to be able to deal with relationship issues in calmer, more rational ways. At the same time, they learn to become aware of their own centers. What works for them? What are their core beliefs and values? Can they openly and gently communicate this personal information? I have seen and personally experienced the true and honest responses that others grace us with (as opposed to emotional outbursts) when we are able to communicate from our authentic selves.

This learning and growing process, both individually and as a couple, is the really inspiring part of exploring the whole area of alternative relationships. The true gift of working consciously with intimate relationships is that it allows one to grow at a very deep, profound and above all wholly satisfying level. My hope, therefore, is that this book will be helpful and inspiring to anyone interested in forming aware, conscious, sustainable and fulfilling relationships.

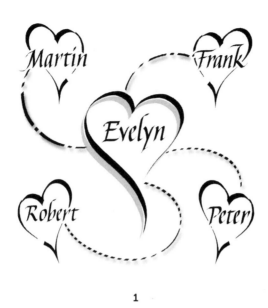

1

Multiple Loves — Evelyn

*Y*ou're young, single, and have a number of boyfriends and it seems like you just *can't decide to settle down and form a long-term relationship with any of them. The thought of "marriage, two children and a house in the suburbs" is simply not something you contemplate without feeling a bit queasy. One of these days maybe, or then again, maybe not. Anyway, for the moment you're enjoying a life of freedom. You're concentrating on your successful career, you feel good about yourself and you have an active social and love life. As time goes by, however, you notice that more and more of your friends are deciding to form committed relationships, or are starting families. At parties, you're often the only single person, and when the holiday season comes around it's difficult to find other people who share the same lifestyle. The pressure from others to settle down or start a family is increasing.*

Evelyn totally understands what this feels like.

Evelyn is a twenty-nine-year-old, university-educated woman who works as a country manager for a large multinational company. She often travels abroad, and she enjoys the cultural diversity that her job provides. Evelyn is intelligent, self-aware, and independent. She enjoys meeting people and quickly feels at ease in new situations.

As a student, she enjoyed a varied and stimulating sex life. Although that particular aspect of her life is somewhat calmer now, she still enjoys her freedom.

Evelyn relishes a great social scene; and she likes to spend time with a few different lovers. There is thirty-four-year-old Martin, the guitarist in a rock band that Evelyn used to sing with. Martin is a close friend. He often comes by Evelyn's house, guitar in hand, and after sharing a lovely meal they play a few songs before spending the night together. Being with Martin is always fun, as they share the same sense of humor and often find themselves doubled up with laughter. Their lovemaking is also full of fun, creativity and pleasure. After Martin stays the night, they enjoy a leisurely breakfast, and bid each other farewell. Martin is fiercely independent and that suits Evelyn perfectly as, in addition to Martin, there is Frank.

When Evelyn is with Frank she feels at peace. Evelyn's relationship with Frank is deeper than the one she shares with Martin. Frank shares her passion for spirituality, and they meditate together regularly. Frank works for a charity and he finds Evelyn's drive, energy and directness inspiring. Frank and Evelyn also have a sexual relationship and sometimes they spend weekends together. They often go for walks in the woods and engage in long, deep conversations before spending intimate evenings together. They both have a sense that they are important parts of each other's lives.

One of Frank's friends recently took his own life, and this deeply affected Frank. Evelyn was an enormous comfort to Frank during this difficult period. Sometimes she simply spent time with him in supportive silence, other times they conversed about his feelings. Through all of this, Frank felt much closer to Evelyn and one day, not long ago, he suggested they live together.

Evelyn's reaction to Frank's suggestion was not what he had expected. Evelyn was not at all keen on the idea of living together. In fact, she made it clear that she might never be interested. She told him that she was very happy with her single life in her own city apartment, and she appreciated the level of contact she and Frank savored at the moment. Evelyn really loves Frank and enjoys being with him, but she didn't want to say no to her life as a single, and especially not to her other lovers. Besides, in addition to Martin there's Robert and Peter, who she sees from time to time. Evelyn also didn't want to exclude the possibility that she might meet other interesting people. Frank was deeply disappointed. He had expected that sooner or later Evelyn would want to settle down. He told her that he thought she was afraid of committing and that she probably had "commitment phobia."

When Evelyn heard the expression "commitment phobia," she started to feel a sense of uncertainty. Was Frank right? Is she only thinking about herself? Maybe she is incredibly selfish? Why can't she, like so many other people, decide to have a long-term, committed relationship? Frank is unique and wonderful, and she really loves him. Is she normal? Maybe she is too demanding and too egotistical? She felt guilty and confused. Would it not be better to simply try a long-term relationship with Frank? With all of these questions, Evelyn decided to give Leonie, the relationship coach, a call.

Commitment phobia

At first glance, it may seem logical to think that someone who "wants everything" and doesn't want to commit to only one partner is suffering from a fear of commitment or "commitment phobia." What exactly is commitment phobia?

Commitment phobia is a relatively new term for a psychological condition where someone has an irrational fear of entering into a long-term relationship. If those who have this condition are already in long-term relationships, they often wonder if the chosen partner is "the right one." They exhibit signs of attraction and repulsion: sometimes convinced that they have found the right partners and want to spend their lives with them; other times confusion and doubt have the upper hand and they retreat. He or she can't be with the same person for too long, and sometimes a long holiday together is too much to handle. Often, socializing with friends comes at the expense of those they love. They form relatively casual relationships, avoid real intimacy and keep their acquaintances from getting too close. People with commitment phobia are often afraid of "melting together" with someone else. They often find it difficult to be completely open with other people or to allow anyone to see their weak points. They're afraid that their own identities are not strong enough and they are afraid that they'll lose themselves, or that they will lose control if they get too close to someone else. The root causes of an inability to commit are often found in the past, a time when the individual didn't experience enough safety to allow the ability to emotionally bond with others to develop.

During my counseling sessions with Evelyn, we first looked for any signs of an inability to commit. We created a retrospective, schematic view of her life and explored the different threads that run through it. On a sheet of paper, Evelyn drew four evenly spaced vertical lines to divide it into columns. Each column represented a seven-year period of her life from birth until the present (ages one - seven, eight - fourteen, fifteen - twenty-one, twenty-one to the present). We then created four rows that helped us to look at the following threads of her life during the different periods:

THE BIOLOGICAL THREAD: the state of Evelyn's health and wellbeing
THE DEVELOPMENTAL THREAD: her educational and personal development
THE EMOTIONAL THREAD: her predominant feelings and emotions
THE LOVE THREAD: details of her love life, her boyfriends and lovers, using drawings of different colored hearts

As she filled in the chart, Evelyn saw that she had not experienced any particularly significant traumas in her life. Loving parents raised her in a warm and supportive environment where they encouraged creativity and independence. There was one incident of note however: as a young child, Evelyn was hospitalized after breaking her leg in a playground accident. The six weeks in a plaster cast had been a trying time for her, as patience had never been her strongest trait. Various projects and visitors helped her during her hospitalization, and she learned to be patient; but this was definitely one of the most difficult memories from Evelyn's childhood.

Evelyn also sees that she is inquisitive and loves to learn. She remembered that she had always finished her homework quickly and would have enjoyed even more assignments. Her development thread indicated that she is always growing in one way or another, both as a child and as an adult. Evelyn always looks for new challenges. She has fond memories of a carefree childhood surrounded by friends, and noted that she was often the one that organized activities. This trait continued to express itself during her college years when she was chosen to be the president of her class. When she left home at nineteen and moved into student housing, she seized the opportunity to explore her sexuality. She remembered how wonderful it was to experiment and to experience the differences between lovers.

Evelyn's love thread contained a noticeable amount of detail. She laughed as she drew many hearts that represented all the men that she had enjoyed time with during her college years. She couldn't remember how many there were; she was simply crazy about sex and really enjoyed it. Later on she drew the hearts that represented Frank and Martin significantly larger than the others she had drawn, and these bigger hearts really stood out. When she spoke about them, her expression changed. Martin kept appearing in her life. It wasn't that she sat around waiting for him; it was just that if he called her on the phone, her heart skipped a beat. She told me that she enjoys being with him because he makes her happy. When they played in the band together they were very close. In fact, she realized now that she had been in love with him. The connection between them changed when she started a new job. Her position required a great deal of travel abroad, and she could no longer sing in the band. Martin has never stopped being in her life though. They always manage to get in touch with each other, and the connection is deep and intense when they do meet. Still, after each rendezvous, they both go their own ways. There is no "must" or "should" about their relationship; they simply enjoy each encounter. Martin and Evelyn are both completely content with their relationship as it is.

Frank is a different story altogether. Evelyn met Frank four years ago at a weekend meditation course. They'd clicked from the moment they met. She told me that she feels safe with Frank and that she feels peaceful and calm when she is with him. In many ways they have a relationship that makes sense to both of them. Frank projects a calm and relaxed disposition that acts as a healthy balance to Evelyn's enthusiasm and drive. Frank is much more serious than Martin.

The crucial point, though, is that Evelyn really doesn't want to contemplate a life without either one of them. She has known both men for so long that they seem to be part of her life now. She feels attached to them — emotionally and physically.

Besides her relationships with Martin and Frank, and her less frequent but thoroughly enjoyable trysts with Robert and Peter, Evelyn enjoys going out for an occasional evening all by herself and, if she meets a man that she feels attracted to, she has been known to invite him back to her place. She likes the excitement of meeting a new man and the sexual exploration that sometimes results. Through our sessions, it became clear that Evelyn prefers multiple partners and, most importantly, different ways of relating with each of them.

As we worked through the drawings, we discovered that Evelyn has no problem being fully open and honest with her partners. She chooses to spend quality time with each of them and gives them her full attention when she does.

Interpersonal connections

One way to become clearer about a relationship between two people is to examine the connections that they have with each other. One of the first things that people do when they get to know each other is to find out what they have in common. If there are areas of mutual interests or experiences, friendships, romances and partnerships can arise. Connections can be divided into at least ten different categories:

1. EMOTIONAL connections express themselves as aspects of trust, safety, mutual respect, values, intimacy, openness, pleasure, caring, humor and a sense of togetherness.

2. PHYSICAL connections are specifically bodily and/or sexual. These connections can take the form of touching, stroking, playful contact, cuddling, kissing, intimate touch and lovemaking.

3. RECREATIONAL connections can be common hobbies or things that are enjoyable to do together. Examples might be athletics, theater, playing cards, making music, etc.

4. ECONOMIC connections refer to the sharing of economic resources. Common examples include being part of a shared household economy and/or living together.

5. FAMILY connections are people who have a blood or a marital relationship, or people who have chosen to adopt or have children.

6. SPIRITUAL connections are experienced by many people as a sense of energetic awareness. This can be a purely personal understanding of connection to one's own inner being, to others, to nature or to a higher power or consciousness.

7. INTELLECTUAL connections occur when people share similar conceptual interests, especially when they can learn from, and creatively challenge, each other.

8. PASSIONATE connections are created between those who share enthusiasm for a common goal, product or creation. Often, each person inspires and encourages the other to reach toward these goals or to bring the product or creation into being. Passionate connections are often found between people who support causes such as finding cancer cures or healing the environment.

9. CULTURAL connections occur between people who are part of the same or similar group. People who make cultural connections often have common beliefs and feel comfortable with a shared set of traditions and behaviors.

10. ESTHETIC connections happen when people enjoy a shared sense of beauty and form in areas such as art and design.

Many intimate relationships are primarily based on emotional and physical connections. When people are also living together, there will most often be economic connections as well. Sometimes there is an additional connection between two people based on specific personalities or character traits, and this extra piece makes the relationship feel special.

Additional connections are quite often why we fall in love. A particular person might have certain qualities or aspects that are important to us at a crucial moment in our lives. For example, we may be feeling a longing to express the artistic side of ourselves, and all of a sudden we meet an artist that inspires us deeply. A powerful passionate and/or esthetic connection might occur as a result, especially if other connections such as emotional and physical attractions are also present.

The qualities and aspects that are important at any given time, however, are not only dependent on personality and character, but also on our development and growth as individuals. What is important to a student might not feel relevant when that person becomes a parent, and so on. The types of connections that we need are not constant and will change over time. Relationships change to reflect this.

The connections that can be found between two people in any kind of relationship, intimate or not, are many and varied. Most people make clear distinctions between intimate relationships and platonic friendships, and use the presence of physical intimacy to determine this. However, there are people who are attracted physically, and who enjoy the other's company, but who don't have many, if any, other strong connections with that person. On the other hand, there are people who have a deep and loving relationship with no physical connection, although they love each other very much. So not everyone has clear distinctions between an intimate relationship and a friendship, and not all people share the same understanding of the boundaries between friendships and deeper connections. This means that some people feel very threatened if their partners form emotional connections with someone else, while for others it's physical connections that spark jealousy. There are also people who don't have a clear sense of their own boundaries. One of the keys to a successful relationship is to find out how we feel about our relationship definitions and boundaries, and to find out what our partner(s) feel as well.

Evelyn and I explored the different connections she feels with each of her boyfriends. We first made a list of what connections were important for her, both in the past and in the present. We came up with the following:

PASSIONATE
PHYSICAL
EMOTIONAL
RECREATIONAL
INTELLECTUAL
ESTHETIC

We then examined her connections with each man. We did this by creating some "connection wheels" on paper. To create a connection wheel, we draw a circle and divide it up into pie sections. Each section represents a type of connection and the relative importance of each one.

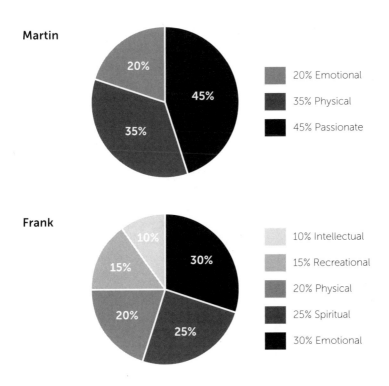

Martin

20%
45%
35%

20% Emotional
35% Physical
45% Passionate

Frank

10%
30%
15%
20%
25%

10% Intellectual
15% Recreational
20% Physical
25% Spiritual
30% Emotional

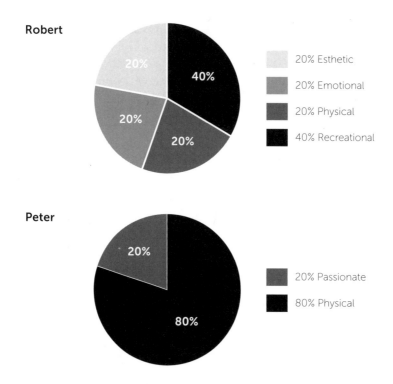

Robert

20%

40%

20%

20%

- 20% Esthetic
- 20% Emotional
- 20% Physical
- 40% Recreational

Peter

20%

80%

- 20% Passionate
- 80% Physical

When Evelyn created these wheels and talked about them, she felt much more sure. When she saw that she is connected in many different ways to each man, she realized that she is actually fully in touch with herself and her own needs. She realized that by creating varied connections, she is fostering the optimal circumstances for her own development and growth. It is wonderful that each one of the men challenges her in his own special way. She also enjoys each relationship for its uniqueness. For her, the physical connection that she feels with each of them is something natural that simply happens all by itself. It would feel very strange for her to deny or suppress the physical attraction she feels for each of them.

Martin, Robert and Peter are fine with this arrangement, but Frank is becoming uncertain. The longer she and Frank know each other and the more intense the contact becomes, the more Frank has difficulty with the fact that Evelyn enjoys sex with other men. Frank is considering starting a family, and a spouse that shares her bed with other men is not something that fits into his picture of family life.

Intimacy and commitment phobia

Someone who has commitment phobia often experiences problems being intimate. Intimacy occurs when we open ourselves to another person, and allow ourselves to be vulnerable. To do this we need to feel safe and be able to trust. The capacity to receive is crucial when it comes to allowing intimacy to occur. To be intimate with someone else, we need to be capable of self observation and self reflection. If we can fully accept ourselves, it's easier to express ourselves to another person.

Intimacy involves the capacity to love the other person, and the capacity to feel that — even when we allow this person to really see who we are — he or she loves us too. To be intimate means being open enough to create a connection. Someone with commitment phobia lacks the confidence, security, and trust that he or she needs to be truly intimate.

Evelyn is very good at creating intimacy in her relationships. She has an open and honest picture of herself including her expectations and boundaries. She was fully capable of providing emotional support to Frank when his friend died. She does not run away from difficult situations. Evelyn does not have commitment phobia; it is just the opposite. Evelyn is able to commit to many people and can love many people at the same time, each in distinct ways. She loves Frank and she loves Martin. She also strongly values her relationships with both Robert and Peter.

Polyamory and Friends With Benefits

To have the life you want,
you have to release all the ideas
that are holding you back.
— ANNEMARIE POSTMA

"Polyamory" and "Friends With Benefits" are new terms coined in the past few decades. They are very useful when discussing modern, intimate and loving relationships. Polyamory (many loves) refers to the capacity to love more than one person at the same time and, just as importantly, the ability to maintain more than one intimate relationship. These intimate relationships can be sexual in nature, but don't have to be.

For most people the word "friend" would not normally be used to refer to someone who they have sex with. However, there are people like Evelyn who have friends that they also enjoy sex with from time to time or "friends with benefits."

The creation of these terms, and the redefinition of some old ones, reflects change in our society. For example, "monogamy" used to mean "until death do us part" with one partner. Now, it simply means one partner at a time. Indeed, many of the terms we use to talk about interpersonal relationships are undergoing similar redefinition. It can be quite difficult to draw a clear line between the concepts of acquaintances, companions, friends and partners. Each relationship is unique and each has its own set of connections. Many relationships simply defy simple definitions.

So, the terms we use to define relationships are changing, and they can mean different things to different people. To avoid confusion and enhance communication it can, therefore, be very useful to talk to our partners about how we view our relationships and the different people in our lives. This creates clarity and transparency and ultimately can help build trust.

Exploring the different connections with her various partners was a real eye-opener for Evelyn. She now understands how she structures her relationships, and that there is nothing wrong with her at all. She has gained insight into why she doesn't want to live together with any one partner. Evelyn's lifestyle works for her.

Evelyn discovered during our talks that she is polyamorous. She loves two men who are both incredibly important to her. In addition, she loves a few intimate friends. She had read about polyamory before but it never seemed relevant to her own situation. As she spoke of this, I asked her one of my favorite questions, my "wonder question." "Imagine," I said, "that all of a sudden a wizard appeared in front of you and created your ideal world — a place where people related to each other as you would like them to relate. What would that world look like? How would people interact with each other? What does love and friendship look like in your world?" I gave Evelyn the task to fantasize about her ideal world in the period before our next session.

When Evelyn returned two weeks later, she was clear: In her ideal world there would be more people like her and not mostly couples and families. There would be communities of people where each person had their own place to retreat to, but also common spaces where people could gather. In her ideal world people didn't make a big fuss about sex but instead felt free to enjoy sexual encounters without having to feel guilty. Their partner(s) would be accepting, encouraging, and happy for each other. In her ideal world, people would treat each other lovingly and at the same time gently challenge each other.

As a result of her fantasy, Evelyn realized that it is important for her to find other people that have similar relationship views. She identified three goals by the end of the sessions. First, she would have a conversation with Frank about her relationship ideals and the way life works for her. At the same time they would explore whether there was some way that there could be a future for them. Secondly, she made plans to search for other like-minded people, not only for support, but also to share her views.

✦ ✦ ✦ ✦ ✦ ✦ ✦

How can women and men come to terms with the discrepancies between what they hold true for them, and what "everyone else" thinks is right? How do we deal with situations such as Evelyn's where we are asked to behave in ways that simply do not match up with our own inner sense of righteousness? At least part of the answer to this puzzle may be found when we understand that societal ideals for right relationships vary from culture to culture, sometimes radically so.

THE NA AND INTIMATE RELATIONSHIPS

The Na, known as "Mosou" in Chinese, live around beautiful Lugu Lake in the foothills of the Himalayas. They are a matrilineal society where the Mother is held in great regard. The Na favor a system of "visiting marriages" where the men leave their homes to visit the homes of their partner(s). Traditionally both men and women could have multiple partners.

Interestingly enough, there is no word for "jealousy" (or for that matter "rape") in the Na language. Relationships are based on mutual affection and when one or both of the partners lose interest, the relationships end gracefully.

One American scholar who recently visited the Na noted "the Na undeniably preserve a gentler culture than our own. Suicide is rare and murder unheard of."

It is worth reflecting on the fact that a society where women (and men) are free to have multiple partners without shame or approbation turns out to sustain a kindlier, gentler people.

Questions you might ask yourself

+ How intimate and open do I dare to allow myself to be with others?
+ What connections do I feel I have with my partner(s); my friends?
+ How do I view myself?
+ What is important for me?
+ Am I free to have feelings and thoughts? Do I dare express them?
+ What would my ideal relationship world look like, and how would people treat each other in it?

Tips for managing multiple relationships

+ Make time for yourself on a regular basis. It's important from time to time to take a break and reconnect with yourself. This will make it easier to fully connect with another person.
+ Prioritize quality time over quantity time. In other words don't fill up your personal calendar, and make sure you stay within your limits. You can only use your time once.
+ Be honest about your expectations and goals in each relationship. It's best to be up front and check each other's expectations explicitly.
+ Be prepared to take risks. Be aware that starting a relationship is risky: You court the possibility of being hurt. You might fall out of love, or the relationship could change — or end. If you have more than one relation-

ship then you increase the chances that you might have to say goodbye to your lover — or that she or he might say goodbye to you.

- Dare to be yourself. Other people feel it when you are unsure of who you are, and who you allow yourself to be. They will often react to this in a negative way. It's much better for you — and others — if you simply don't cater to uncertainties and concentrate instead on who you are. It's simpler that way.

- Pay attention to your partner(s) and let your partner(s) know how important they are to you. Make time for each other. Be efficient and practice time management.

- Make clear and straightforward agreements with each other, and stick to them. Reevaluate your agreements regularly and see if they still work for both of you, or whether they need to be modified. Every individual and every relationship evolves, and needs change over time. By reevaluating regularly you can avoid difficulties.

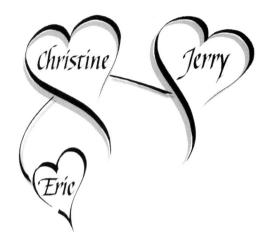

2

An Impossible Love — Christine

You're married, have children and you are in love with someone else. You've always thought it was terrible when you heard about this happening to other people. You never thought it could happen to you. Until one day you realize… you're in love! All the signs are there: the butterflies in your stomach, the daydreams, a new surge of energy in your life and exciting encounters with your new love. At the same time you're suffering as your feelings of guilt and shame increase each day until suddenly — panic! What do you do now? How can you deal with these feelings? You don't want to choose, you can't choose, and you are afraid you'll lose everything.

This is the overwhelming state that Christine found herself in one day.

Christine, thirty-two, is married to Jerry, forty-two, and they have two young children. Christine and Jerry first met each other at a local community association meeting. Jerry had been in the middle of a messy divorce at the time and had poured his heart out to a sympathetic and attentive Christine. Jerry is a quiet, introverted man of few words. He's a hard worker, honest to a fault and totally reliable. Jerry had a conservative Protestant upbringing, which is evident in his attitude toward the father's role in family life. He and Christine get on well and they have a terrific family.

Christine loves Jerry very much, and she is very aware that she made, and continues to make, a conscious choice to be with him. Jerry is certain, honest and steadfast, and he has always provided Christine with a feeling of security and safety, which she continues to value very highly. Christine has a hard time making decisions, and Jerry provides her with a grounding counterpoint.

Still, Christine finds it difficult to talk with Jerry about things that are truly important to her, especially when it comes to her own feelings. She has tried to talk to him at various times over the years, but he usually responds in a way that puts her off because he shows little authentic interest. He doesn't seem to understand why she makes such a fuss of things. Everything is OK in their lives isn't it? They've both got work, the family is healthy and happy, what is there to talk about? Christine feels like Jerry simply doesn't understand her. As a result she has, over the years, slowly stopped trying to talk to Jerry about herself. The children require more attention as they get older and it seems like the easiest thing to do is focus her conversations with Jerry on the kids. The truth is that, like Jerry, Christine had never really learned how to talk about her feelings, so it is very easy to simply avoid the subject. This state of affairs seemed to work for both of them — until the day Christine met Eric.

Eric is open, extroverted and communicative; and when they met at work one day, the two of them hit it off at once. Eric is curious and inquisitive and he wanted to know everything about Christine when they met. They often went for walks and talked and talked and talked. Talking seems to be incredibly easy for Eric, which is a real contrast to Jerry. When Eric asks questions, he doesn't give up until he gets to the bottom of the issue, and he is prepared to really listen. After many walks and conversations, Christine found herself opening up more and more to Eric. It didn't take long before Christine realized that she was developing feelings for him. Eric had already admitted that he thought Christine was wonderful and said if she hadn't been married to Jerry he would have been very interested in exploring a relationship with her.

It has become more and more difficult for Christine to ignore her feelings for Eric. She really looks forward to their lunches together and she often finds herself thinking about him. She managed to keep her feelings to herself until one day, not long ago, one of her colleagues mentioned that she was looking uncommonly happy. All of a sudden, Christine understood what was going on: she was in love! She was shocked when the reality finally sank in. She tried to make it simply go away, but thoughts and feelings about Eric kept returning.

Christine didn't dare say anything to Jerry about what was happening. Jerry's ex-wife had cheated on him for many months and when Jerry finally found out, well, that was it. There was no discussion or attempt to save their marriage. Cheating is, for Jerry, a non-negotiable issue. Jerry is still very angry with his ex, and has very little contact with her. Jerry is adamant: he will never allow this to happen to him again. Jerry's view is that you choose a life partner and you commit. Falling in love with someone else is, according to Jerry, something that destroys families. Christine feels devastated as it appears that she is now creating exactly the same situation that Jerry's ex-wife did. Christine knows that telling Jerry about Eric would mean the end of her marriage and she doesn't want that. So, she simply doesn't know what to do.

From time to time, Christine dreams about having a family with Eric. Sometimes she doesn't even recognize herself when she is with Eric, he's so different from Jerry. At the same time this worries her. Her greatest fears revolve around the consequences for her children. She does not want to subject them to the trauma of a divorce. She's already seen the ramifications of Jerry's divorce, and life is not easy for the son from Jerry's previous marriage. In fact, Christine has never been able to understand how Jerry's ex could have cheated on him. Truthfully, Christine thinks that Jerry's ex-wife is self-centered and egotistical. How could this woman have risked her family for her own selfish needs?

She now struggles with her incredible feelings of guilt and she feels like she is an awful person to be doing such a thing. Her internal emotional battles are raging, she is losing a lot of weight and she's sleeping badly. There simply doesn't seem to be a way out. At this point Christine gives Leonie, the relationship coach a call to see if she can help.

Falling in love with someone else

In my coaching practice, I see countless situations where a client has fallen in love with someone other than his or her partner, and becomes completely confused. Some of this confusion stems from love's accompanying strong emotions. The greatest source of turmoil, however, is often the fact that many people are afraid of their own reactions to what is happening. They react differently than they thought they would. In short, the picture that they have of other people that cheat does not correspond with the picture that they have of themselves. All of a sudden they find out that they have the same longings and sometimes are even acting the same way as other people that have affairs do — the very same people who they might have judged harshly. This is a powerful internal confrontation and it can be very disturbing.

Many times when people fall in love they don't immediately realize what has come over them, and it is difficult to make rational, considered decisions about how to proceed. When they're in love, their view is distorted by a hormonally induced haze and they may not be able to fully comprehend the consequences of their actions and decisions. It's only when the biochemical rush of being in love subsides, and an inner sense of discernment reasserts itself, that a realization occurs that some self-evaluation is necessary. This is exactly what happened to Christine. She suppressed her feelings and convinced herself that not talking about it made it less real. It's only when a colleague pointed out that Christine had changed that she realized what was happening — that she was in love. Help!

People in our society tend to be critical about falling in love with "someone else." Monogamy is still the norm and is something that the majority of the Western population subscribes to, often without thinking about it. Most people, when asked what the ideal relationship looks like will answer, "two people in a long-term, committed, monogamous partnership." Still, for many people this doesn't work. In the Netherlands, forty percent of the population cheats or has been cheated on, and thirty-five percent of marriages end in a divorce. In about a third of these divorces, marital infidelity is cited as the reason for the breakdown. In the United States, between forty and fifty percent of all marriages end in divorce; and seventeen percent of all the divorces that occur are reportedly due to infidelity by one or both partners concerned. This figure is probably higher because many states do not recognize infidelity as grounds for divorce, so although cheating might be the actual reason for the breakup, it goes undocumented. Studies undertaken by Atwood and Schwartz in 2002 show that forty-five percent of married women and forty-eight percent of married men engage in extramarital affairs at some point or the other. Clearly, infidelity happens and is happening. Yet, consistently more than ninety percent of adults questioned in both countries still consider infidelity a bad thing. So, many people are doing things that the vast majority of the population find unacceptable, and as a result there is a lot of judging going on!

Christine knew all about judging those who cheat; she did it herself. She has seen the sorrow and pain infidelity causes; she has seen families torn apart and has observed the difficulty for all concerned; she has judged Jerry's ex particularly harshly. And yet, here she is, in love with someone else! She is experiencing first hand how incredibly difficult it is to manage emotions, as she judges herself. How could she look her husband in the eye anymore? What has become of her?

Understanding feelings of guilt and shame

For many people the first step in trying to make sense of a difficult situation is to try to think clearly about it. But in a situation such as Christine's, this is difficult as there are strong negative emotions that make it hard to think straight — guilt and shame. Understanding these feelings, and where they come from, can help us to deal with them.

Why do we feel guilty? Well, most commonly, we find ourselves in situations where we're convinced that we cannot live up to either our self-expectations or other people's expectations of us. Our expectations are built on the norms (behaviors) that we think are correct. These norms are connected with certain values we hold, and are often based on what we've learned as children. Christine, in this particular situation, values honesty, and the relationship norm that correlates with honesty is faithfulness. Christine believes in life partnerships. There is no room for anyone else. Feelings of guilt arise, then, when we discover through new circumstances or new situations that our internal desires, or indeed our actions, are no longer in alignment with our norms. We no longer measure up to our own expectations. Christine believes strongly in being faithful and her feelings of love for Eric appear to be in direct conflict with this. It's no wonder she feels guilty.

Feelings of guilt are often accompanied by anger, usually because we feel that we aren't strong enough to adhere to our own internalized set of norms. When we feel anger, often time it is a sign that we've overstepped some kind of internal boundary. Something has happened that shouldn't have happened, and yet it did.

In Christine's case, her self-directed anger probably indicates that she needs to allow her internal desires to come into sync with her norms. In other words, Christine needs to find a way to allow her feeling of love with someone else to somehow come into alignment with her need to be faithful.

Synchronization can happen in two ways: we can either change our behavior to match our self-expectations, or we can reexamine our norms. For example, Christine has, indeed, fallen in love with someone else, so she could simply stop being in love. Unfortunately, Christine feels that she has tried this and has not succeeded.

One way to explore the other alternative, reexamining our norms, is to ask ourselves some questions. What do the norms that we have accepted in the past look like now, based on our current experiences? Would we like to modify them? We might notice a need to do this and we might even notice that the norms that we had in the past were formulated too rigidly. For Christine, this might mean her concept of being faithful might be modified to allow a complementary relationship, if Jerry could know about it and accept it. That of course, given Jerry's values, is a big "if."

So we may sense a need to adapt our norms, but modifying our own norms will not help us to deal with the expectations of our partners, or of others such as our families and our friends. In Christine's case, she realizes that she shares Jerry's norms when it comes to life partnerships and having strong feelings for others outside their relationship. She now understands that her sense of guilt also comes from the fact that she feels that she is not living up to Jerry's norms either, and she feels like a failure as a result.

Feelings of shame occur, therefore, when we judge ourselves not only for our own desires, but also for our thoughts about how others perceive us. This judgment is often brought out by others but, ultimately, it is our own. If we feel shame, it's very hard to look dispassionately at what has happened and it's difficult take a good hard look at what our individual roles are. When we feel shame, we often feel tendencies to retreat into ourselves. So feelings of shame can lead to passivity. This is where feelings of panic can arise as we are tossed between wanting action and at the same time wanting inaction, or to hide. So what to do? There seems to be no way out of this dilemma, and that is exactly what Christine feels — stuck.

Acceptance

Forgive yourself for not being at peace.
The moment you completely accept your non-peace,
your non-peace becomes transmuted into peace.
Anything you accept fully will get you there,
will take you into peace.
This is the miracle of surrender.
— ECKHART TOLLE

Being in love, feeling love or even feeling affection is natural and, in principle, is a good thing. We admire and are attracted to someone else for what he or she is, and there is nothing wrong with this. It's just a feeling. An important way of coming to terms with feelings of love for someone is to simply accept our feelings. They are what they are, and we feel what we feel. Trying to deny certain feelings doesn't solve anything. Even worse, the more we try to suppress our feelings, the stronger they become. If something is not allowed — it's exciting! So, the more we tell ourselves that we're fools for having fallen in love, that it's all wrong and that it's not permitted, the stronger our attention is drawn to these forbidden feelings. If, on the other hand, we relax and accept the feelings they will often calm down. Anyway, it's not all negative. When we fall in love, even with someone outside our partnerships, it can bring movement and growth both within our relationships and within ourselves. If handled well, falling in love, no matter with whom, can be a tremendous positive force in our lives.

Self-compassion

Self-compassion — the ability to accept ourselves for who we are — can also be a powerful way to accept our feelings.

Compassion, as we know, means that we acknowledge that someone else is having a difficult time. We feel, as it were, their pain and we want to help or support the other person. We are gentle and understanding towards the other person and their imperfections. We understand that the other person can make mistakes, as they are human and thereby imperfect. We also understand that what has happened to them could happen to us. We feel warm and caring, and are prepared to release any judgments.

Self-compassion is nothing other than having compassion for ourselves. It's the ability to look at ourselves with love and respect, especially when we fail or make mistakes. Instead of criticizing or judging ourselves, which is usually our first reaction, we view ourselves with softness and gentleness. We give ourselves all the support we require. We accept that we are just like everybody else with shortcomings and areas to develop and grow. We accept ourselves completely for who we are, even when we don't live up to our own expectations or match our ideal pictures of ourselves. Mistakes happen, as do feelings of frustration, loss, pain and having overstepped our own boundaries. That's all part of being human.

Whether we expect it or not, falling in love happens too. We need to try to allow ourselves to enjoy our feelings, instead of feeling guilty. Feelings of love and affection are best left to simply flow through us, whether or not we give any concrete expression to them.

We can choose to do something with these feelings, but ideally our choices are made by consciously taking into regard the wishes of our partners, and by respecting any agreements we have made with each other. It can be good to look at those agreements from time to time and verbalize them for clarity's sake. This can only happen if we summon the courage to speak about our expectations, promises and agreements openly. Of course, it is possible that we don't know what we want to do — or not to do — with our feelings. In such cases, we can try to give ourselves the time and space needed to explore and understand them before making any hasty decisions.

Exploring being in love

Everyone, whether they are conscious of it or not, searches for inner wholeness. An intimate relationship offers an ideal manner to grow in the direction of wholeness. Being in love can provide the same opportunity.

Being in love says a great deal about us, and where we are on our developmental paths. When we meet someone who has a quality that is missing in ourselves, we are often attracted to them. Other times, we're attracted to someone who embodies something we recognize, or someone who notices us. We feel affirmed because they truly understand us as we share similar qualities. All of these are aspects of an underlying truth: often, we are really in love with our ideal selves, or with our own character traits that have not been expressed fully.

Everybody grows and develops over the years, and it makes sense that occasionally, we will meet someone that triggers awareness of our underdeveloped sides. We can see this when we look at Christine's situation. Being open about her feelings is not something Christine can do easily. Being more communicative and forthright is something she has always wanted to work on. It's not something that Jerry necessarily encouraged over the years, because he has similar tendencies, so Christine gradually shut down until eventually she stopped trying. However, when she met Eric, this inner desire to express herself openly and freely reasserted itself. In many ways, Eric acted like a messenger that brought a cry from Christine's unfilled need. For example, Christine really likes it when Eric questions her, and then won't accept "I don't know" for an answer. She has the feeling that he is really interested in her inner world.

In the meantime, at home, Christine has become quieter and quieter. Jerry has noticed this, but never persists with his questioning, as that simply isn't in his nature. He does his best to comfort Christine by offering an extra hug from time to time, or he puts a cup of tea in front of her. Christine is glad that Jerry leaves her in peace but she is secretly somewhat disappointed. Does Jerry really not see that something is up? Eric would keep asking....

During one of the coaching sessions with Christine, we took a look at her relationship requirements using *The Relationship Game* from Peter Gerrickens. We identified her top ten important needs for her relationships. *The Relationship Game* consists of fifty cards, where each card has a relationship ideal printed on it. I asked Christine to imagine what her most perfect relationship would look like, and to choose cards that reflect correlating characteristics. We then placed the cards into three groups, one group for needs that were met by Jerry, one group for needs that were met by Eric and one group for needs that were met by both men. When we looked at the "Relationship Cards" that Christine chose and sorted, it became obvious that her essential needs were pretty evenly spread across both of her current relationships. The relationship with Jerry fulfills her desire for shared caring and fostering of their children, offering practical assistance, maintaining a sexual relationship and showing love and affection to each other. Both relationships fulfill her desire to have fun together with someone. The relationship with Eric fulfills her requirement for supporting each other emotionally, encouraging and challenging each other, giving compliments and valuing each other, sharing feelings with each other about personal issues and surprising each other. Soon Christine exclaimed, "Oh, if I could glue these two men together! They both offer things that I find important in a relationship."

Taking personal responsibility

Normal life can be a prison,
until you accept responsibility for yourself.
— ANNEMARIE POSTMA

In her heart, Christine blamed Jerry for the fact that he is not open, doesn't speak with her and doesn't show his feelings. She felt that Eric made her much happier because he is curious, interested in her and challenges her to express herself. I asked Christine how she makes sure that her relationship needs are met in her marriage. Christine discovered that, when it came down to it, she was not being open to Jerry. Christine realized that, "come to think of it," she didn't know what was "going on inside Jerry's head or heart at all." This means that she cannot, from her side, offer him any emotional support as, quite frankly, they really don't talk to each other very much. Christine also discovered that she does not express her needs clearly to Jerry and has not asked him about his needs. As we talked, Christine began to become aware of the part she plays in the behavioral patterns they have created in their relationship.

For Christine, though, one point became absolutely clear: even though she would love to express her feelings for Eric, she does not want to cheat on her husband. She also wants to get rid of all the fantasies and daydreams she has about Eric and a future with him. During our conversations, we examined her dilemma in depth by laying out all the possibilities Christine had available to her, including the positive and the negative consequences of each of them. What would it look like if she chose to be with Eric? What would it look like to stay with Jerry? Would it be possible to talk to Jerry about the fact that she was in love with someone else and make room in their marriage for a relationship with Eric?

Making choices

Uncertainty is fantastic glue.
It leaves you stuck to where you are.
— OLAF HOENSON

Choosing to do one thing is inextricably tied to the fact that we choose not to do something else. It's therefore important to accept that when we make choices, they can sometimes carry negative consequences for us and for others. In other words, someone is bound to be disappointed. Examining negative emotions and recognizing and accepting them is work that many people would rather not do, but it can be an enlightening process. It takes a lot of emotional energy to resist the negative aspects of a choice. We can free up energy if we allow ourselves to accept and feel the pain and sadness a choice can bring with it and let these emotions simply wash through us. The moment we truly accept a feeling is the moment it becomes lighter. We can give ourselves the time to process our feelings and then focus on the possibilities available to us.

Freeing up energy to make choices happen

When we need to make large, life-changing decisions it can be very helpful to find someone who will listen without judgment. Someone who does not have a vested interest in our choices can look at a situation in an unbiased fashion. Sometimes it helps to literally step back from the situation by taking a few days to go on a retreat, vacation, or to take long walks in nature. Solo hikes, or chatting with people who don't know us, or even reading inspirational texts can often bring new insights and clarity.

During our sessions, Christine realized that she needed to make a choice. Although emotionally she would have loved to create space in her marriage for a complementary relationship with Eric, she knows that this was simply not something she could ever talk to Jerry about. If she did indeed choose to be with Eric, she was very afraid that it would be a real battle to sustain a good relationship with Jerry and the children. She simply did not want to take that risk. She had made a conscious choice to be a mother, to have a relationship with Jerry and to continue down that path. She has always loved, and still does love Jerry, and in many ways they have a good life together. She realized that she needs to learn how to talk with Jerry about her feelings as well as his and, in any case, she wants to share some of her new insights with him.

Through coaching, Christine began to learn how to open herself to Jerry and how to express herself more clearly to him. She learned how to give constructive responses and how to speak more directly using "I" statements. She discovered that when she tried these techniques, Jerry reacted much less defensively. This improved their communication. At the same time Christine, as a result of her understanding that she does not want to cheat on Jerry, has moved to a new division in her workplace and has broken off contact with Eric. Although this has been tough for her, she feels better, and anyway she feels that Eric deserves a woman who can be there fully for him and who he can start a family with. She cannot be that woman, as her place is with Jerry and their children. Christine also attended an assertiveness course where she learned to be more true to herself. She never did tell Jerry about the fact that she had fallen in love with Eric. The true gift of the experience, despite the inevitable sadness and grief that she feels for the loss of her relationship with Eric, is that she has learned how to more fully invest her energy in the relationship that she has ultimately chosen.

THE THREE GODDESSES

For many women, a sense of who and what they are constitute crucial elements in their life-choices. In the West, women often use terms such as student, employee, daughter, wife and mother to define themselves. Many traditions around the world, however, have different views of women based on the idea of The Three Goddesses. These goddesses, whether Celtic, Hindu, or Greek, have connections with the moon phases, agricultural seasons and, most crucially, the stages of a woman's life. The most common terms for these stages are Maiden, Mother and Crone.

The Maiden is a young girl with all of her attractiveness and beauty. The Mother is the caregiver and nurturer. The Crone is a woman who has moved into her power, wisdom and grace and who fully owns and expresses her sexuality. The understanding is that all women contain these three Goddess elements at all times, but, usually, one or the other surfaces during any given period.

Our Western culture glorifies the Maiden, and accepts the necessity of the Mother, but rarely, if at all, values the Crone. A pervasive example of this can be seen daily in media images that depict sexually attractive women as young, thin and impossibly proportioned "maidens." Where are the beautiful mature women in all of this? Ancient Taoist manuscripts reveal that in the past, the most respected bearers, transmitters and teachers of the age-old Sacred Sexual traditions were women in their 80's and 90's! Almost all pre-patriarchal cultures have references to older, experienced women who were deeply respected for their wisdom and learning.

Despite negative contemporary images, mature women are choosing to step into their Crone power, and nowhere is this more evident than in relationships. For many women, serving and caring, whether in a family setting or otherwise, is simply not enough. The need to be a whole person and the desire to continue to learn, create, and express themselves cannot be ignored. This need for growth and integration sometimes, unfortunately, conflicts with the rigidity that Western societies have created in the realm of interpersonal relationships.

What of the woman who wants to explore the totality of her being within a long-term, sustainable relationship? Not all relationships can accommodate this, especially if they are based on rigid, nonnegotiable roles and boundaries that tend to cater to the giddy joy of new love that the Maiden might experience, or the solidity, stability and security that the Mother provides. Relationships that negate flexibility, openness and a commitment to mutual growth can lead to a woman having to make, at times, painful choices. The good news is that more and more people are exploring alternatives to traditional role-based relationships that do, indeed, make space for exploration, discovery and authenticity — characteristics that also hallmark the Crone goddess.

Questions you can ask yourself if you fall in love with someone else

+ How do I see myself when I am in love? What judgments do I have (if any)?
+ What does being in love tell me about my relationship needs? What are those needs?
+ How do I take personal responsibility for my relationship(s)?
+ How do I make choices for the future?
+ What are the repercussions of my different choices?
+ Will my decisions create new problems? What are the long-term consequences?
+ How will my family be affected by my choices?
+ What am I most afraid of?
+ What does being in love mean to me, and to my relationship?
+ What is the state of my current relationship?
+ Can I talk with my partner about being in love with someone else?
+ Are there things missing in my current relationship that I can't get from my partner? What does the new person I am in love with offer me that my partner can't?
+ Is this the first time I feel attracted to someone other than my partner?
+ Can I give myself permission to look openly and honestly at my feelings for this person and what my feelings signify?
+ What makes this other person different? What does he or she have to offer? Why is he or she so special? How can I develop that special quality in myself?

Tips for being in love with someone other than your partner

- ACCEPTANCE - Accept that you are in love and accept the feelings that accompany it. It is nothing to be ashamed of. Stop resisting. If you accept your feelings, they will not intensify nearly as fast as they would if you try to suppress them. Allow yourself to enjoy them.

- STAY IN BALANCE - Falling in love with someone is a great time to make sure that your existing relationship(s) are in balance. Be honest with yourself and with your partner(s).

- EXAMINE YOUR VALUES AND NORMS - Take a look at your values and norms when it comes to intimate relationships. If they change when you are in love with someone other than your partner, reevaluate your self-expectations. Decide if you are being truthful to yourself.

- MAKE CONSCIOUS CHOICES - Think clearly about what you want to do. Avoid being seduced by short-term thinking like "it's only once, I'm sure this is OK." Consider the long-term consequences and balance your choices carefully.

- DISCUSS OPENLY - If you keep all of your thoughts to yourself, you create distance between you and your partner. Dare to talk about your feelings, but be careful with the way you describe yourself. Sometimes it helps to first talk things through with a friend to allow strong emotions to subside.

- DON'T PROCRASTINATE - If you've made a decision, then take action. The longer you wait, the more difficult it can be. Certainly consider in advance what other people's reactions might be, but don't let that paralyze you.

- TAKE TIME - Give all people concerned time to get used to the new situation. Avoid making decisions based on strong emotional responses. If the emotions are too strong, take some time out or talk about the situation with an uninvolved third party.

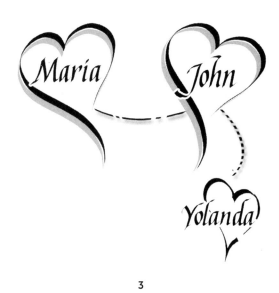

3

I Couldn't Help It:
Recovering From An Affair —
John and Maria

She is young, single and full of life when you meet her; and you think she is amazing. She is very interested in you too, and you both do not hesitate to start flirting like mad. You love it. You feel seen again. She really enjoys the attention and the excitement too, and the flirting moves up a notch. Your e-mails and text messages give your days new dimensions. Pretty soon she asks you around to her place after work. There's a new assignment that needs some extra attention. You decide to take a chance and call your wife, tell her you'll be home late. You go to your colleague's apartment and, sure, one thing leads quickly to another. In the back of your mind you know that you are crossing a boundary with your wife, but you want this woman so much, you want all of her right now.... So begins a period of enjoyment, sexual pleasures and lust — and cheating.

After thirteen years of marriage, Maria discovered that John was cheating, and their relationship was seriously threatened.

John and Maria first met fourteen years ago, when John was thirty-six and Maria was thirty-five. They both had been frequent daters, but very soon they realized that this was not just another short fling, this was something special and more serious. It turned out that the start of their relationship marked the beginning of a new phase in both of their lives. They moved in together quite soon after they met, and their children were born shortly afterwards. They made some agreements before deciding to start a family, one of which was that they would always talk to each other if either of them found themselves sexually attracted to someone else. Neither of them believed that this would happen though, as they had already partaken their fair share of sexual experiences, and neither felt a need for further explorations.

During the first years of their marriage, John was barely aware of other women. All of his attention was focused on his relationship, his career, the new house and their young children. This changed, quite unexpectedly, the day Yolanda appeared.

Yolanda is an attractive, intelligent and vivacious new colleague that joined John's department six months ago. John responded with great fervor when Yolanda showed sexual interest in him soon after they met. Somewhere deep inside himself John knew that something wasn't quite right, but the attraction between him and Yolanda was very strong. All of a sudden, John's agreement to talk with Maria about such an eventuality seemed to have been made in some other lifetime. John had great difficulty keeping his feelings in check and, to be honest, he didn't want to. He wanted to enjoy the excitement between himself and Yolanda. He had missed this so much!

When Maria and John decided to live together, John's work was quite demanding and required him to work very long hours. If he was free in the evenings he often went to the gym or he was busy at the computer. Maria felt, therefore, that she bore the brunt of the responsibility for the household. After the birth of their first child she had reduced her working hours to part-time, which was easily done as she is a nurse. John, on the other hand, was really focused on his career and there was no way he could work part-time without jeopardizing his position. They made a joint decision that he would continue his full-time job and she would be responsible for the care of the children.

In the beginning of their relationship, John and Maria enjoyed an exciting and fulfilling sex life. After the children were born, however, their sex life slowly changed. They made love less and less often, and when they did have sex they didn't spend a great deal of time at it. This wasn't a problem for Maria. She was really focused on her role as a mother, and to be honest she couldn't be bothered with sex as she had neither the interest nor the energy for it. Often, she simply let John get on with it even though she wasn't very interested. Her reasoning was that at least he would be satisfied. Unfortunately, he wasn't.

Maria discovered completely by accident that John was cheating. She walked past his computer one Friday morning and happened to read an e-mail from Yolanda to John, which he had left open when he rushed off to work. The content explicitly showed something going on between John and Yolanda. Maria was perplexed. She thought that they were happy with each other and their family life but now it seemed that, at least for John, this wasn't at all the case. Anyway, hadn't they made an agreement to discuss such things? Of course, infidelity can happen in any marriage, but they had promised to talk with each other and to work out a way to deal with such an occurrence. Now, just the opposite has happened! Apparently, John has something going on with this woman, Yolanda, and he hasn't so much as said a peep to her. Maria felt deceived, and she was furious. The carefully constructed life that she had invested so much in was all of a sudden crashing down around her.

Maria confronted John with the e-mail that evening. To start with, John was incensed. How dare she read his private e-mail! Didn't he have a right to some privacy? Finally, the truth came out: he and Yolanda had been having an affair for over two months. It was purely sexual and there was nothing else to it. Maria was the woman of his life, they had children together and he wants to stay with her; but she simply wasn't there for him when it came to his need for a fulfilled sex life. He was a healthy man, quite frankly, and he needed a bit of sex in his life. Yolanda could willingly offer this and, to be frank, Yolanda really enjoyed it. He couldn't say that about Maria!

Maria felt betrayed. She was very disappointed and incredibly upset. Her partner had cheated on her, and she was being blamed for it! She was outraged. All weekend, they barely spoke to each other, and the following week Maria focused all of her attention on the children. Maria talked about what had happened to some sympathetic friends while John threw himself into his work and let off steam at the gym. At bedtime they avoided each other as each one crept to opposite sides of their bed.

It took over a week for John and Maria to get to the point where they could speak to each other and talk about what to do with the situation. John apologized profusely and explained to Maria that he had let Yolanda know straight away what had happened. He had explained to Yolanda that their affair needed to stop immediately as things were completely out of control and he was in danger of losing his family. Maria was unsure. She didn't know how to carry on with their marriage. How could she could ever trust John again? Yolanda still worked in the same office as John did, right? Wouldn't he see her every day? How could Maria be sure they weren't still at it? What had happened anyway? How often had Yolanda and John met, and where? Did she really want to know all the details? Maria knew she wanted to stay married to John, but had no idea how to accomplish this. Above all, Maria felt incredibly suspicious and mistrustful of John. In the interim, John confirmed that he and Yolanda had agreed to permanently end their affair, and that Yolanda had promised not to try to rekindle it. This was not enough to reassure Maria; and she was still deeply upset with John's deception. They muddled on in this unhappy state for a few weeks until Maria decided that they needed outside help and called Leonie.

The consequences of cheating

Cheating, infidelity, affairs, secret liaisons… call it what we will, throughout history people have engaged in sex without fully disclosing it to their partners. For the purposes of this book, we use a very specific definition of cheating: it's when someone breaks a relationship agreement with his or her partner and has sexual or physically intimate contact with another person. Sometimes the agreements that are broken are clearly and explicitly made between the partners, but more often than not they are based on unspoken and many times little thought about assumptions. The most common assumption is this one: If a relationship is serious, then it must be monogamous. Monogamy, for better or worse, is still the norm for long-term relationships in most Western cultures. In addition, the belief that serious equals monogamous is strongly reinforced when two people fall in love and focus all of their attention on each other.

This belief in monogamy is not reflected in our behavior, however. Recent surveys confirm that anywhere between twenty percent and sixty percent of all adults in Western cultures involved in supposed monogamous relationships have either cheated or been cheated on at least once. In other words, at least one in five, and possibly as many as three in five, consenting adults have experienced infidelity. So there is no question that people do have sexual attractions outside their committed relationships, and yet this is not something we easily speak about. Indeed, admitting extramarital attraction is something that most people avoid doing for fear of the consequences. So when it does happen, most people try — at great cost to their integrity — to maintain the facade of monogamy.

Many times, cheating is a sign that there is something in a relationship that needs attention. In this case John has certain needs that are not being adequately met in his relationship with Maria. Their sex life, as is so often the case, was put on the back burner when their children were born. They've never really taken the time to sit down to talk about this dramatic change to their relationship and events have now overtaken them.

In my practice, I often see the consequences of breaking a relationship agreement. Cheating erodes trust, and it's no simple task to restore it. When we have been cheated on by our partners, we often find the lying and the dishonest behavior far more painful than the actual infidelity or even the fact that our partners harbor feelings for a third person. It can be even more hurtful if we are met with systematic denial when we ask questions that are based on strong suspicions. In fact, cheaters often react by throwing these questions back at their partners and accusing them of mistrust or of causing difficulties. For the one who has been cheated on, this compounds the pain when they subsequently discover that they were right all along.

We often have feelings or an intuition when our partners are having affairs, and we often notice that something is up long before there is any concrete proof. We notice the small details and sometimes there is an uneasy feeling that something doesn't quite stack up. Often, we don't dare to listen to our intuitive hunches because of the unpleasant consequences that can arise when the truth is finally revealed. Sometimes it seems safer to simply set our suspicions to one side and carry on as if nothing has happened. At least life can go on as usual… until the moment when the truth can no longer be ignored. At that point, all the puzzle pieces fall into place, and the true picture is revealed.

Dealing with the aftermath — not all advice is useful

It's an incredible shock when we discover that our partners have been lying to us over extended periods of time. For some people, discovering an affair means the end of the relationship. The pain is so great and the trust so badly broken that splitting up seems like the only option. This is often the initial reaction that is based on strong, overwhelming and seemingly uncontrollable emotions. All of a sudden, life is turned upside down. Everything we've created together over the years seems to have been built on an illusion. Nothing is the same anymore, our world is in tatters. Our partners are no longer the people we thought we once knew. And there's the rub. Everything is unsure: can we ever trust them again? The honesty and security that we thought we built our relationships on has been destroyed.

Sometimes it helps to talk to close friends, but not always. In any case, they may not have much to offer other than sympathy. Friends and family will have reactions based on their own emotional responses and experiences and they may be giving us well-meant but ultimately biased advice. Despite the fact that they are coming from a place of love and caring, their advice may not lead to a solution that really suits us.

Take time

One of the most important things we can do when we have discovered that our partners have cheated is to give ourselves time. Wait until the worst emotions have settled and try not to make hasty decisions. People can go their separate ways at any time — there is no need to rush. If a couple has children, then it's important that the parents stay connected with each other. For the children's sake, if nothing else, it's important to maintain a good relationship with each other. We want to be sure that the children's need for love, safety, support, appreciation and acknowledgement are met no matter what is happening to their parents.

If we are overwhelmed by negative emotions such as sorrow, anger and pain it is very difficult to arrange things satisfactorily for our children. In other words, we need to try to differentiate between the role of a partner and the role of a parent. If we can learn to do that, especially when children are in our presence, it can make a huge difference. All children, and especially young children, need to know that they are not at fault when their mothers and fathers are unhappy or angry. Sometimes it makes sense to tell the children that we need to take a little time to work out some difficult situations that have nothing to do with them.

It is completely normal to experience feelings of disbelief, anger, bitterness, sorrow and loneliness when we discover that our partners have cheated on us. Sometimes it can even feel impossible to focus on anything else as our energy is totally consumed by what has happened. Dealing with feelings of betrayal is, in most cases, a time-consuming process, so it helps if we can allow ourselves the space to let our emotions take their course. If we can do this, we also create room to decide what we really want, and how we want to go about it.

On the other side the of coin, if *we* are the cheaters then it makes sense to take time to truly recognize and understand the consequences of what we have done. It often happens that the decision to cheat is made very quickly, sometimes in a fraction of a second when we are under the influence of powerful hormones that have been released into our bodies. When our partners discover what has happened we are suddenly confronted with all of their pain and sorrow. This is usually extremely difficult and upsetting to see. Our guilt feelings can be so overwhelming that they obstruct our abilities to acknowledge and understand what has happened, and to fully comprehend how we could have let our deception go so far. It can also be really tough to figure out what exactly we want to do now that it's all blown up.

It can be useful if both partners listen to their inner needs and express them to each other during this time. For example if strong emotions are getting the upper hand and we can't find a way to talk with our partners, it can help to agree to a cooling-off period. We might find a close friend to visit for a few days, or spend some time at a place of retreat.

Eventually, the injured couple will need to decide whether they both still want to continue their relationship, and if so, how. At the end of the day, there is no way to avoid this discussion. Sometimes it helps to talk outdoors during a long walk, or in a public place where there are other people present like a restaurant, or a café. Sometimes, it feels like we just can't manage to have the discussion at all. In such a case, it can help to talk to someone like a coach or a counselor who has no vested interest in our relationships and can view the situation dispassionately.

Getting clear about relationship objectives

When Maria and John came to see me, it quickly became evident that they were both very interested in continuing their relationship, but that they lacked the tools and skills to sort out their situation. They were simply going around in circles and getting nowhere. Talks with friends had brought a bit of clarity and consolation but not enough new insights to allow John and Maria to go forth in a healthy direction. In my experience, their stated desire to stay together was a good starting place. If a couple has a real commitment to each other and to their relationship the success rate increases dramatically.

When both partners decide they want to continue their relationship, they also need to agree on how to go about it and where they are headed. In other words, they need to have common objectives regarding both the process and the goal. In my practice, I see many partners that have very different relationship objectives. Sometimes they both say they want to stay with each other, but one of the two doesn't dare say what he or she knows in his or her heart: that it is all over between them. This is quite often the case when he or she feels they have done everything they can to save the relationship. For them, going to relationship counseling is often seen as a weak last effort. In my experience, there is little point in coaching if someone lacks a heartfelt commitment to the relationship. The most common result is that the doubter stops coming after one or two sessions, and ends the relationship anyway.

Making the explicit commitment to stay together often establishes a good first step. I put the "wonder question" to John and Maria to do just that.

The wonder question

The "wonder question" is a tool that I use a great deal in my coaching work. Remember? It works likes this: Just imagine for a moment that a good fairy (you might imagine someone like Glinda, The Good Witch of the North from the *Wizard of Oz*) appears in front of you with a magic wand. This is no ordinary magic wand, but a special deluxe version that really can bring anything into being, such as your most daring fantasy, massive positive changes that you might want in your life; or that your most amazing plans will come true. In other words nothing is impossible for your good fairy. The wonder question method is a good way to bring suppressed desires and wishes up to the surface and to talk about them.

I asked John and Maria to use the wonder question to fantasize their answers to the following questions: If you could magically fix your situation, what would you do? What would your relationship look like a year from now? What would the rest of your life look like? What would have changed? What would you be doing differently? Close your eyes, concentrate on your questions and think about how you would like to magically change your life if the good fairy could change everything. Let obstructive and/or blocking thoughts such as "of course, in reality that can't happen" or "my partner would never accept that" simply melt away. Imagine that the good fairy can do anything, even the impossible.

After Maria contemplated the questions for a while, she told me that in her future she would still be together with John and the children. He would come home more often, work less hard and be more engaged with the family. She would be able to trust him and their sex life would have blossomed again.

John said that in his desired future scenario, he is still with Maria and the children. Maria would complain less and they would have more time to do things together. Their sex life would be what it was like before they had children. They would spend more intimate time together and Maria would enjoy this as much as she once did. John also imagines he and Maria doing more sexually exciting things together. He fantasizes that they might make love outdoors or experiment with other activities.

As John and Maria listened to each other's wishes they recognized, on the one hand, a shared desire to continue their relationship; and on the other hand, a gap to overcome. John blames Maria for losing interest in sex, and Maria blames John for not being honest. They're still stuck.

Effective communication

Better to light a candle, than curse the darkness
— CONFUCIUS

Blame is probably the most ineffective method of communication that exists. The only thing blame usually accomplishes is further separation. Attempting to establish who is the guilty one makes it very difficult to find a solution or to identify needed changes. It's better to focus on the process of acceptance — starting with accepting the pain and sorrow that is. After that acceptance, we can look into the requirements that are under these emotions such as needs for consolation, patience, honesty and trust. By doing this, we focus our attention on the present and the future. We can't change the past, but we can learn from it.

Good communication is one of the most important success factors in a relationship. How do we communicate well? In intimate relationships, there are three important, interrelated skills that can help with good communication: Active Listening; Acknowledging Your Partner; Speaking Honestly.

Active listening

Listening seems simple. All we have to do is sit down and keep quiet while someone else tells us something. Easy, eh? Actually, nothing is further from the truth. Listening — *really* listening — is one of the most difficult elements of good communication. Most of the time, as we listen to someone else, our own responses and reactions to what is being said are forming in our minds. The moment this starts to happen we are no longer fully able to listen to what the other person is saying and so we are no longer really hearing them. Before we know it, we start to defend ourselves and we start to explain that, no it wasn't like that, it was like this. We try to put the other person in the wrong, to convince them that we are correct, or we start giving them advice. These are all very human responses, but ultimately they are quite counterproductive.

Active listening is more than simply hearing the person's words. Instead, it involves focusing completely on the other person and trying to totally take in, and ideally understand, his or her point of view. We are, as it were, trying to see the world through the other person's eyes and to feel what he or she feels. When we practice active listening, we put our own thoughts to one side and allow ourselves to be open to whatever the other person is experiencing — whether we like it or not, agree or disagree, know more, etc. We then reflect what we have heard without interpretation or additional commentary. We don't respond or dialogue; we simply give the other person the chance to verify that we have heard them accurately. If we haven't got something right, they can clarify or repeat what they've said until we (and they) are sure that we have, indeed, heard accurately.

Most people are not used to actively listening, but it is something we all can learn to do. Practice makes perfect, and this does take practice.

Acknowledging your partner

When we learn how to listen accurately, and let our partners know that we have heard them correctly, an important outcome can occur: the person feels acknowledged. Acknowledgement is what happens when our partners know and, just as importantly, feel that they have really been heard. This acknowledgement is more than just letting them know that we have precisely heard what they have said, it lets them know that we accept that they have their own points of view. What they are saying doesn't have to be right or wrong; it is simply what they are saying, and we accept that they have said it.

John tried the active-listening exercise with Maria. He sat quietly and listened carefully when she described what she felt when she found out that he was having an affair with Yolanda. He didn't interrupt and he paid attention to the exact words she used. When it was his turn to reflect back to Maria, he said: "I understand that you were incredibly shocked when you found out about Yolanda and me and that you were angry and upset. It hurt you deeply that I was not honest with you and you are afraid that you will never be able to trust me again." The way he said this to Maria, without defending himself, meant that Maria felt completely acknowledged. She was allowed to own her feelings — her sorrow and her loneliness were given the space to be.

Maria then had the chance to listen completely to John. She reflected back to him: "I hear you saying that you're very sorry that you were not honest with me. You blame yourself and you feel like there is nothing you can do to make things better. You're doing your very best to give me and our relationship positive attention and you find it very difficult that I am responding in such an inconsistent fashion. Sometimes it seems like everything is OK with me and then sometimes I'm angry and upset. You feel like you never know which Maria you're going to have to deal with at any given time. That makes you unsure. You would really like to move forward but you simply don't know how, and you really don't like the idea that you will be having to say 'I'm sorry' for the rest of your life."

As John and Maria learned to listen honestly, openly and accurately to each other they started to understand each other much better. The pain that each of them felt started, albeit slowly, to soften and subside.

Speaking honestly

The third skill that can make communication effective is learning to speak honestly. This means being open to each other; not only about how we feel and how we have experienced things but also about our wishes and our expectations. To speak honestly requires two things: courage and vulnerability. We often find it difficult to express what we really want and wish. We are afraid of other people's reactions, and sometimes pride gets in the way.

Many of these fears are based on one primary fear: the fear of rejection and thus the fear of loneliness. If we let our fears dictate our behaviors, we will never be able to give ourselves the chance to manifest what we really want. Instead, we sabotage ourselves. If we are serious about improving our relationships' (and indeed our own) development, then we will need to gather the courage to accept our vulnerabilities and to communicate honestly with our partners. By learning to listen actively and to acknowledge our partners, we create the safe conditions to be open and honest.

So how do we discover what our wishes and desires are? One way is to simply think about them a bit. In my practice, I use *The Relationship Game* to do this.

When John and Maria played *The Relationship Game* together, they discovered that they have some relationship requirements in common when they chose cards for: Love And Affection; Share Care And Fostering Tasks; Enjoy Things Together; and Take Into Account Each Other's Wishes And Needs. As we talked our way through the different cards, we discovered that the words on the Sharing Care And Fostering Tasks card carry very different meanings for John and Maria. Maria wants household chores to be done her way. She is often quite critical of John, and tends to nag him because he keeps house differently than she does. These are often seemingly minor things like the way he folds up clothes or towels. Also, on the one hand, Maria criticizes John for not engaging enough with the children; while on the other hand, she scarcely gives him a chance. He doesn't enjoy this at all, since he has a need to be valued and complimented instead of being blamed for being inadequate. As a result, John withdraws, goes to the gym more often and comes home later and later. Maria then feels like she's being left to do everything on her own and blames John even more. They each play a part in the creation of this negative response circle.

> *When you point a finger at someone,*
> *take a look at your own hand*
> *because there are three fingers pointing back at you!*
> —ANONYMOUS

The most important thing to do when we want to break out of an unwanted relationship pattern is to find the answer to this question: What can *I* do to break this circle? It's always much easier to expect our partners to be responsible for making changes in our relationships. However, when we give the control to our partners, we give away our power and make ourselves dependent on someone else. It can be much more constructive, therefore, if we take responsibility for our own actions and have a good hard look at what *we* might do differently. It can be a good idea to consider whether we want to take into account other peoples' needs as well. If we do, we can ensure that we make constructive changes in our behavior.

When John saw the negative circle he and Maria are stuck in, he admitted that, ideally, he would like to stop retreating when Maria comments on what he does, or doesn't do. He also wants to take more initiatives when it comes to taking care of the children, and he would like to stop conceding every time Maria tries to step in and take over. For her part, Maria would really like to be less critical of John and the way he does things around the house, and she'd be happy to let him do things his way. She would like to learn how to be a bit less controlling. It turns out that this has been a life issue for her, even before she met John — a revelation that reassures John. Maria would also like to give John more compliments and to show her appreciation more often. John and Maria both discover through this exercise that they share the same intentions and that these intentions are important for both of them.

Some of the other cards that we looked at in depth were: Be Faithful To Each Other and Maintain A Sexual Relationship. John and Maria had already understood that when their children were born it seemed like all of a sudden Maria became a mother at the cost of everything else. John likes the fact that Maria is happily immersed in her activities with the children but he does miss the intimacy she once shared with him. He mentioned this to Maria, but she simply dismissed him. "The children need time and energy and there's always tomorrow" is her standard reply. The truth is that she has no energy or desire at the end of long days to engage in a serious lovemaking session. If he is really frustrated, she suggests he take care of himself. For her that is the end of the discussion about their sex life.

It was not the end of the discussion for John though. He pointed out that he doesn't want Maria to do anything she doesn't feel like doing so he never pushes the issue. But he does feel rejected and frustrated. Maria feels less and less accessible to him. If John wants to hug or kiss her she pushes him away, as she is afraid that if she responds it will lead to sex. So not only is there less sex, but the reduction in hugging and physical contact means they are generally less and less intimate.

Sexual relationships and the passing of time

It is very common that the way we have sex as well as its role in our lives changes as our relationships mature. There's an old Dutch story that says that during the first years of a relationship couples should deposit a coin into a jar every time they have sex. Later on, when they've been together for a few years and their sex life has begun to slow down a bit they can change their system and start to withdraw a coin each time they have sex. It turns out that at the end of a long life together, they will end up in balance, as the rate of deposit is much faster than the rate of withdrawal. This story shows that there is an accepted understanding that it's normal that the frequency of sex slows down over the years. There is a biological explanation for this: after a while the creation of "falling in love" hormones in our bodies diminishes and is replaced by "bonding hormone" production. Our relationships change emotionally and intellectually as well. After we've lived together with someone for a while, life begins to settle. We begin to know how each other works, we become familiar with each other's foibles and other parts of our lives demand attention such as friends, our social networks and hobbies. The arrival of children is always a turning point in a relationship. Although we've got nine months to prepare ourselves for the birth, it's not really possible to totally foresee the changes.

Children require love and attention, which takes some getting used to and requires us to make adjustments. Many men find it quite difficult to see their partners change to become, primarily, mothers. The attention and love that one partner gives to the other is suddenly shared. Usually, a mother has already bonded with her child during pregnancy and experiences a strong connection with the baby when he or she is born. It is not at all uncommon for fathers to feel somewhat excluded during this time, even when they feel prepared for the baby's birth and love their new child.

Furthermore, a relationship can seem self-evident, or taken for granted, especially when there are children that are perceived as a "glue" that binds a family together. Therein lies the danger as our relationships will usually suffer when we take them for granted. It is important that we not only take time to parent but to also make time and energy for our roles as intimate partners.

John and Maria felt the repercussions of not focusing attention on their relationship. John understands Maria's role as a mother, but he has real needs as a partner in a relationship, and he's looking to Maria to fulfill them. Maria enjoys intimacy with John but often follows that sentiment with a "but...." Maria now realizes that this is causing problems in her relationship and she is working on accepting more and controlling less. She's working on softening her perfectionism, and now encourages John to take on some of the family responsibilities.

They've arranged for childcare one evening a month so they can go out together. For his part, John is listening much better to Maria and is no longer firing back his own solutions when she speaks. They are now doing their best to be more present for each other, and since Maria is no longer quite as tired, they have started to make more time for intimacy between them. They've seen the impact that these conscious changes have had on their relationship, and they are finding it easier now to talk about their sex life and what they might do to enhance it.

When sexual desire is mismatched

You can't bake bread in a cold oven
—ANCIENT CHINESE SAYING

Generally, most women need significantly longer to warm up than men do during lovemaking, particularly if they have been in the relationship for a long time. It can take only a few minutes for most men to become fully aroused whereas the average time for most women is between fifteen and twenty minutes. It is quite surprising how few couples take this into account when making love. Another significant difference between the sexes is that most men enjoy direct genital contact during foreplay, while many women enjoy non-genital stroking and massage. Therefore, one way for a man to increase his partner's satisfaction is to learn some patience! The more a man can learn to focus on gentle, relaxing and non-sexual contact, the greater the chance that they will have a mutually satisfying sexual encounter if it happens. For many people, non-sexual touch is very important as it creates a sense of safety and connection, and Maria is no exception in this regard.

There are many ways to make sure that both partners have the environment they need to be fully present during sexual activities. One of the simplest — and yet for many couples surprisingly difficult — things to do is to reserve time and space for their lovemaking. It can be very rewarding to have planned non-sexual activity first — such as a massage. The idea is to create an undisturbed space where sexual energy can naturally flourish in an environment that nurtures it. Two sexual myths tell us: "if people love each other sex will just happen,'" and "desire is always present." It doesn't, and it isn't. We have to work at it.

John and Maria have now decided to set aside time once a week, when the children are out, to be intimate with each other and this has improved their sex life dramatically. Still, John sometimes longs for the excitement that he experienced with Yolanda. By this time John and Maria have improved their communication skills as well as their level of trust to the point that it is possible for them to talk about this in a relaxed and open fashion.

A brainstorming session can be a great way to explore possible ways to give our sex lives new energy. To be successful, we should strive to adhere to a few brainstorming rules:

- Think only in terms of possibilities. Both partners are allowed to say anything, and nothing is wrong, even if the idea in question seems crazy, bizarre, strange or undoable.
- As different possibilities are mentioned, list them on a piece of paper. This is a good way to uncover secret fantasies and to come up with new ideas.

It's only when all possibilities have been named that the process of seriously considering which ideas are feasible and which are not is started. A brainstorming session is also an excellent way to rule out — in a lighthearted and relaxed way — things someone might not personally be interested in.

John and Maria bounced a few ideas around during a brainstorming session on the topic of spicing up their sex life:

- go ahead and have a fling, but don't tell the other person about it
- accept that the other person has a friend with benefits
- go to a swingers club together
- attend some type of intimacy course together

After the brainstorming quieted, they looked at the pros and cons of each idea. They decided the idea that they felt most comfortable with is to first invest in their own sexual relationship during the next twelve months. To get started, they agreed to attend a tantra-massage course together where they can learn tools to enhance intimacy between them. They also agreed to reevaluate in six months and check that the agreement is working for both of them.

Sex and love

Many traditions emphasize that sex and love are two very different concepts. In the West, we tend to lump them together, and for many of us the two are inextricably intertwined. In John's case, it's very clear that just because he is sexually attracted to Yolanda doesn't mean that he doesn't love Maria. For Maria, this is very important to hear and to understand.

According to some spiritual teachings, it is of paramount importance to create conscious and respectful situations to work with sexual energy. When John and Yolanda met their sexual energy was high. They both knew that Maria was not aware of what was happening and this means that it was much more difficult for them to consciously and fully express their sexual energy. Some part of them had to suppress or actively ignore the fact that Maria would be deeply hurt if she knew what John and Yolanda were doing, and so they had to block their awareness of this to be able to carry on with their connection. There is no moral judgement attached to this statement, it is simply an observation: if we have to shut down part of our awarenesses, then it's impossible to be fully conscious.

During our sessions, John and Maria learned to become clear about these two areas. They realized that they do still love each other *and* that sex is important for both of them. They also see that it's important to be able to speak clearly and openly about this without blame or judgement and to learn to hear what is important for each of them. By learning to communicate openly and honestly about sexuality, they can rebuild trust. This then makes it possible for them to find ways to create space for conscious sexual energy in their relationship.

SEXUAL ENERGY AND LOVE
IN SPIRITUAL TRADITIONS

Sexual energy is, according to many ancient spiritual traditions, the most powerful energy that we have available to us. It is, after all, the reason for our very existence. It is a driving force behind much of our hard-wired instinctual behavior and the biochemical systems that support it.

Many spiritual traditions teach that sexual energy is dangerous and that controlling lust is a very important part of being a good person. Interestingly enough, many of the foremost representatives of those very same traditions have had sexual relationships while at the same time preaching abstinence and control. Clearly sexual energy is very powerful indeed.

There are, however, spiritual and cultural traditions, both Eastern and Western, that embrace sexual energy and have developed methods of working consciously and openly with this powerful, natural force. Many of them have been ruthlessly suppressed but some have survived and are enjoying a new found resurgence. The most widely known are the Tantric traditions from India and the Taoist Sexual Yoga practices from China.

The Tantric Sacred Sex tradition, often referred to as simply Tantra, originated in India but refers to practices used throughout southeast Asia. Tantra refers to a complete worldview in which the conscious use of sexual energy has an important role as a tool for spiritual development. Incidentally, when we start to explore the world of Tantra in the West, we soon discover that the vast majority of teachers and authors have some sort of connection to the teachings of an Indian self-styled guru called Osho, a.k.a. Bhagwan Shree Rajneesh (1931–1990). One of the difficulties with the term Tantra is that it is often synonymous (in the West) with Osho's ideas about Tantra. There are many different interpretations of Tantra even amongst traditionalists in India and Tibet. Having said that, there are a great number of practitioners and teachers doing excellent work under the banner of Tantra.

Taoist Sexual Yoga has been, until recently, a little known branch of Taoist knowledge. Taoism (Daoism) is an ancient Chinese philosophy that has informed and guided Chinese culture for over five thousand years. Tao (pronounced "dow" and also spelled "Dao") means "the way" or "nature's way." Taoist Sexual Yoga was traditionally considered part of the Inner Alchemy (Nei Dan) practices of self-cultivation. Taoist Inner Alchemy practices are used to promote spiritual development as well as physical health. This dual process of spiritual and physical development is also known as "cultivating original nature and life." Taoist Sexual Yoga focuses on the conscious use of Jing Qi (sexual life-force) for health and spiritual development.

Both of these sex-positive traditions differ radically from the prevailing Judeo-Christian view of sex as something to be feared, suppressed or as a source of shame. As more and more people reject sex-negative paradigms, the traditions from other cultures have proven to be a rich source of inspiration. The idea that sexual energy can be used as a powerful tool for both personal and spiritual development is something that many in the West are finding deep resonance with. Viewing sexuality without shame is a crucial step to regaining our abilities to make informed choices in intimate relationships.

Questions you might ask yourself

+ How do I deal with negative emotions?
+ What are the goals I have either in my current relationship, or in one I would like to have?
+ In what ways do I listen to my partner?
+ How do I acknowledge my partner's feelings?
+ What part do I play in any problems I may have in my relationship and what do I do to break negative circles?
+ What are my sexual needs, expectations, desires and fantasies? Have I talked to my partner about them?

Tips for life after cheating

+ Use a cooling-off period.
+ Make sure you and your partner develop common relationship goals. Determine what new relationship goals, both short and long-term, you might like to create with each other.
+ Be prepared to listen.
+ Acknowledge your partners feelings.
+ Have patience. It takes time to deal with sorrow, anger and pain.
+ Be prepared to learn from the past and to examine the relationship patterns that you have created.
+ Look at the part you play in these patterns, both the individual ones and your overall behavior and attitudes.
+ Have the courage to forgive yourself and anyone else involved.
+ Be prepared to reinvest in your relationship.
+ Work on creating clarity around your own relationship needs and talk about them with each other.
+ Together, reevaluate the agreements you make with each other on a regular basis.

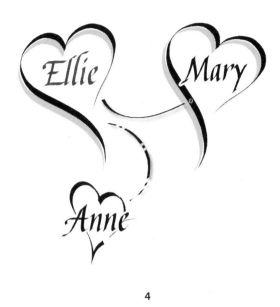

4

A Secret Relationship — Ellie and Mary

*S*ometimes, out of the blue, it simply overwhelms you. You've been happily together with your partner for years, and despite the normal ups and downs, life still is good together. Then one day you get to know someone that makes such an incredible impression on you that there is simply no way to avoid falling in love. What starts with a simple chat and an innocent flirt soon develops its own inexorable tension that leaves room for only one thing: a step further. You don't want to upset things at home, your partner would never understand it anyway and you don't want to cause her unnecessary suffering. So you keep it to yourself. Soon enough there is the first kiss, followed by hugs and exciting text messaging. Then, before you know it, you find yourself having the most amazing sex together. It is so wonderful that you naturally want to carry on. After some time you suddenly realize: I've got a secret relationship. You rationalize away or suppress your guilt until the moment your partner discovers your secret.*

This is exactly what happened to Ellie and Mary.

Ellie, forty-seven, and Mary, forty-two, have been together for eighteen years and have lived together for the last fifteen. Mary is the biological mother of their two children. Ellie and Mary love each other very much. Ellie is an artist, expressive, loves unexpected surprises and is full of life and initiative. She likes to go out, she spends time with the people in her large network of friends and acquaintances and she is always looking for new ways to sell her paintings. Mary works as a teacher, provides a steady income for the family and looks after the household. She is tidy, orderly, enjoys cooking and loves a warm, cozy home. Their very different characters complement each other well and they've had a wonderful time together over the years. There is only one cloud on the horizon — their intimate relationship has diminished from the great passion they enjoyed when they first met. They almost never make love anymore, although they still cuddle a great deal. Mary really doesn't have much of a need for sex and Ellie has accepted that her girlfriend has less of a desire for intimacy than she does. Despite this, Ellie had never considered a relationship involving anyone else. Ellie and Mary have always had a strictly monogamous relationship.

A while ago, Ellie organized an exposition of her work and met Anne, who had provided the catering for the event. Anne is thirty-five and is quite a driven and passionate organic wine entrepreneur. She is single and she was incredibly attracted to Ellie from the moment she saw her. Anne recognized her own drive and passion in Ellie when Ellie talked about her art. After the exposition they both stayed on while Mary went home to relieve the babysitter. Ellie and Anne simply couldn't stop talking with each other. Anne was very impressed with Ellie's paintings and told her that she was simply not commercial enough in her thinking. It seemed like she had hundreds of suggestions of how Ellie could further her carrier as an artist. They got on so well that they decided to help each other out in their respective livelihoods. Ellie offered to introduce Anne's wines to her network of friends and acquaintances and Anne offered to help Ellie make her artwork more visible to the world. They sealed their deal with a kiss. Before they realized it another kiss followed, and then another. The adrenaline and excitement got the better of Ellie and before she knew it she was lost in Anne's arms.

Ellie headed home in a euphoric state after that first kiss with Anne. When she arrived home, however, she realized she had a strong need to spend time by herself. Luckily, Mary was asleep. The following morning Ellie acted as if nothing had happened. She never imagined that it would be so easy to hide something from Mary.

Ellie and Anne stayed in touch. Anne was as enthusiastic as ever and often dropped by Ellie's studio to chat and to float new ideas. Their kissing and cuddling had become increasingly intense and finally, one afternoon, they ended up making love. In hindsight, it seems like there was no way of avoiding it as they had become so close. Ellie got so much energy from her contact with Anne. Not only was Ellie's art career progressing much faster now, but she was more inspired than she had been for years. She also noticed how much she had missed an active sex life and how important sensuality is for her. In the meantime she never said a word to Mary about the nature of her connection with Anne. Ellie didn't want to hurt Mary, and she was very afraid of what Mary's reaction would be. The last thing Ellie wanted to do was to endanger her family situation. The reality, however, was that the contact she had with Anne was too important to stop. Her relationship with Anne was a catalyst for her new journey of self-discovery. Anne was constructively critical and challenged Ellie to stand up for herself, especially in business situations. This was totally different from Mary, who thought Ellie's paintings were nice, but didn't seem to care much whether Ellie was commercially successful or not. Besides, Mary was busy with her own work, the children and the household.

At home, Ellie spoke more and more enthusiastically about Anne. Mary became suspicious that Ellie's relationship with Anne was more than just friends. She finally asked Ellie if there was more to the relationship with Anne than Ellie was letting on. Ellie denied outright that there was anything other than a purely business relationship between them, and that there was absolutely nothing to be jealous about. Where on earth did Mary get such ideas from? Mary was quite upset with herself after this exchange and blamed herself for having so little trust in Ellie. She told herself that she should be happy that things were going better for Ellie. She seemed so much happier lately, and that was really great to see. Still, Mary had a feeling that something was not quite right. When she tried to raise the subject again, Ellie reacted angrily… and so Mary stopped asking questions. She decided that it was all in her head — she'd been imagining things.

When Mary started to ask awkward questions, Ellie discovered that the step from concealment to lying was really quite small. Ellie was again surprised that it was so easy to lie to Mary. She didn't want to hurt Mary and she knew that Mary would be devastated if she told her what was really going on. She loved Mary so much. Still, Ellie's feelings were stronger than her will power, and against her better judgement, she continued to see Anne in secret.

Nothing further was said on the subject — until the day Mary stopped by Ellie's studio unannounced one afternoon. She poked her head in the door and saw Ellie and Anne in a situation that left nothing to the imagination. Anne and Ellie were totally engrossed in each other and didn't even notice that Mary had entered the studio. Mary pulled the door quietly shut and left the building in tears. Once outside her anger exploded. So there it was after all! She'd asked so often and Ellie had always denied it. Well, she couldn't deny it now. She relived, almost like a movie, all the occurrences of the last few months. It all made sense now. How could she have been so stupid and believed Ellie instead of her own intuition?

Once back at home, Mary withdrew into herself and when Ellie came home, Mary said nothing to her. She wanted to wait until Ellie said something herself, but nothing happened. And then, when Ellie said something quite trivial about Anne, Mary could no longer contain herself. She exploded. How could Ellie deceive her like that? Didn't she know what would happen to their relationship? They had a family! What now? How could she ever trust Ellie again? Ellie burst into tears. How could she have told her? She didn't want to tell Mary as she knew how hurt she would be. Of course she didn't want to threaten their relationship. But the contact with Anne is so important for her and for her career. Her paintings are really taking off at last, thanks to Anne!

Mary was too angry and shocked to be able to speak calmly to Ellie. When the children were around, Mary pretended nothing was wrong, but of course the children felt that something was not right. When Ellie and Mary did try to talk, they simply went around in circles and blamed each other. After a few fruitless weeks they decided they needed professional help, and contacted Leonie.

Falling in love and
New Relationship Energy (NRE)

Falling in love is one of the most incredible and intense occurrences we can experience. Our entire view of the world is altered when this happens. Our ability to think clearly and make wise choices is compromised due to a combination of a biochemical cocktail of hormones unleashed into our bodies and the emotional upheaval of New Relationship Energy (NRE). NRE is created the moment we are attracted to another person and it grows in strength as we fall in love and create intimate relationships. NRE doesn't last forever, though; it slowly subsides over the months and years that follow. Life, when you are full of NRE, feels completely different to life in a settled, long-term relationship where the partners know each other through and through. Very often when we are in long-term relationships and then fall in love with someone else, we experience it as something completely extraordinary. It's very common to feel that we've never had this with our partners or, if so, that it was so long ago that the experiences are only vaguely remembered. Ellie experienced all of this when she fell madly in love with Anne. And so, the way the secret relationship between Ellie and Anne started is not unusual.

When we find ourselves in a situation such as this, many of us cannot find the strength to react rationally to our feelings and to what is happening to us. Although many of us who have had affairs say that we couldn't help ourselves, most of us know exactly when we have crossed our own lines for what is right and what is wrong. That's not to say that we consciously choose to cross this line, but that we know in retrospect when it happened. The decision to keep going can be impulsive, but it can also be because somewhere inside ourselves, we have decided that this relationship is so important that we don't want to pass it up. We choose, more or less consciously, to continue. However, this doesn't mean that we always fully think through the consequences for our existing relationships.

From a biological point of view, falling in love has enormous effects on our bodies. The sheer volume of hormones that are released have powerful effects on our feelings and our behavior and it is very difficult to not be affected. Anthropologist Helen Fisher has done many studies in this area and compares falling in love to substance addiction as it affects the same parts of the brain. Most people are aware of how difficult it can be to stop using alcohol, painkillers or other drugs, and dealing with NRE is no easier.

Dealing with NRE

It might sound counterintuitive, but one of the best things we can do if NRE has us in its grip is to tell our partners what is happening. The reason for this is that secrecy and suppression are two things that help NRE to increase in strength. Indeed, throughout the ages, forbidden love recurs as a theme in dramas and tragedies. Consider Romeo and Juliet or Tristan and Isolde where lovers die in each other's arms. Open and honest communication with our partners can free us from the turmoil and internal raging that NRE creates. Often, our partners intuitively know that something is happening anyway. Openness creates trust and understanding, and it can also give us great opportunities to express our emotions and thoughts. This can help us to return to places of balance and peace and can motivate us to make well thought out decisions. When we navigate from a foundation of inner peace, ultimately we make choices that benefit all concerned.

> *Understanding with feeling is not human,*
> *Feeling without understanding is not wise.*
> —EGON BAHR

Five tools to help resist falling in love

Sometimes we simply don't want to fall in love but find it happening despite our seemingly best efforts. Here are five things that we can do to help in such situations:

1. **TAKE RESPONSIBILITY:** acknowledge our own role in creating and maintaining new relationships

2. **EXERCISE OUR INTELLECTS:** use our abilities to think rationally

3. **STAY MINDFUL:** be aware of what we are doing — step back and observe the situation from a distance

4. **USE WILL POWER:** decide what our ultimate goals are and stick to them

5. **BE DECISIVE:** when we have decided to act, act

Some of us know all too well the consequences of allowing ourselves to fall in love with someone other than our partner(s), but lack the willpower and decisiveness to resist our feelings. Whether we can resist them depends partially on our characters and temperaments, but it is also affected by our abilities to act independently. If we're used to making our own decisions, then it is a little easier to avoid simply giving into our feelings and our desires at critical junctures. So there is a direct connection between autonomy and the ability to deal with falling in love unexpectedly.

In our first session, I asked Ellie and Mary to tell me, each in their own words and without interruptions, their sides of the situation that had brought them to my practice. As I listened to Ellie, I understood that she has not fully developed a number of the skills and abilities mentioned above. She simply let herself go at the art show (after drinking a few glasses of "altogether excellent" wine mixed with the influence of a good dose of adrenaline that had been released with the excitement of meeting Anne). Anne took the initiative to kiss her, but Ellie allowed it. Ellie was totally aware of what she was doing and felt a strong sense of responsibility towards Mary and her family, but lacked the willpower and decisiveness to deal with the situation differently. Being with Anne revealed intense feelings that Ellie really missed and that were much stronger than what she knew in her relationship with Mary. Ellie simply didn't manage to think about the long-term consequences of what she was doing. Her common sense deserted her. It just felt so good, and she allowed her feelings to take the upper hand. Ellie put her ability to think rationally to one side, so her willpower and decisiveness (what little she had available) were never called into play.

Broken trust

The discovery that someone has cheated or has been dishonest over a long period of time creates an enormous break in the trust between two partners. Stephen Covey, in his book *The 7 Habits of Highly Effective People*, speaks of a relationship's "emotional bank account" that is funded with goodwill, which has been built up over time. This "balance of goodwill" drops precipitously when the existence of an affair becomes known. Rebuilding this reserve of trust after such a calamitous event can take a huge amount of time, effort and emotional investment.

Ellie and Mary are completely clear that they want to stay together. Neither of them can contemplate the idea of a life without each other, and their family is incredibly important to both of them. To get the process of rebuilding their relationship underway, they decide on a cooling-off period. Ellie agreed that during this period she would put her physical relationship with Anne on the back burner, as long as she could maintain some contact through e-mail and telephone. This was hard on Anne, but Anne displayed both understanding, patience and a willingness to support Ellie and Mary during this difficult period. Still, it was very difficult for Ellie and Mary to move forward. Mary was extremely unhappy with the fact that Ellie had lied to her for such a long time, and found it difficult to think about their future together, or how they could move on. How could she trust Mary again? Mary found it very difficult to forgive Ellie for what she had done.

Forgiveness means letting go of the past.
—GERALD JAMPOLSKY

Forgiveness

We can easily, albeit unwittingly and without warning, find ourselves stuck in similar situations; and like Ellie and Mary, we wish that we could somehow undo the past. When we do this, we resist the reality of what has happened, and this denial takes energy. When we resist reality, we not only lose energy but we also become dependent. When we are stuck in the past we become victims to it and we never take full responsibility for ourselves and the situation.

No matter how much we want to, *we just can't change the past*. What we can do is acknowledge and accept it. Accepting and acknowledging the past releases all the energy we have been using to resist it. We have to accept what has happened before we can begin the process of forgiving our partners.

Forgiving is a difficult step to take, and for many of us it seems virtually impossible. We think that forgiving means we are somehow saying that what the other person has done is OK. We think we're giving the other permission to do what they have done, that we're letting the situation go and telling them that it's no longer important. Forgiving our partners can also feel somehow inconsistent with the pain we feel for what has happened. However, forgiving is absolutely not something we do to make our partners happy or to put them at ease. It's not at all about simply crossing out what has happened and moving on. When we forgive, we are not telling our partners that we are OK with everything that has happened and that their behavior is all of sudden something we are now prepared to condone. So if forgiveness is *not* these things, then what is it?

Forgiveness is ultimately an acknowledgement to ourselves that we are making a conscious decision to no longer let our lives be defined by what has happened. We are choosing to no longer allow the pain and sorrow that has been evoked by a particular circumstance run our lives. When we define ourselves in terms of our pain, we make ourselves dependent upon it. We become in a sense a victim of the other person, and we hand our power over to them. Forgiveness is choosing to retake control of our lives by facing the future and consciously focusing on how we can have a positive influence on today and tomorrow. Forgiveness doesn't just happen though, there are a few steps required.

Forgiveness tips

+ Be prepared to forgive
+ Release any idea that the past can or should be different
+ Acknowledge reality and accept it
+ Make your expectations and disappointments clear
+ Be prepared to adjust or modify your expectations
+ Express and work through your feelings of anger and sorrow
+ Stop any kind of revenge or "getting even" behavior
+ Have compassion for the other person and see the world through their eyes

♦ Develop self-compassion
♦ Receive and accept any acknowledgements from the other person for what they have done

The "See It Through My Eyes" exercise

It is not easy for Mary to move forward in her relationship with Ellie. During my conversations with Mary, it became clear that she is having problems accepting that her notion of "family" is no longer valid now that Ellie is in love with someone else. She's asking herself what's left of her family, of "the four of us together?" Had it been a case of self-delusion all along? Anyway, what had Ellie been thinking? Didn't she consider the effect of her actions on the family? What does their family mean to Ellie? Even if Ellie is physically present, isn't she thinking about Anne all the time? Could she really forgive Ellie?

When I asked Mary what she needs to move forward, it appeared that, first and foremost, she needs to be able to express her feelings. Ellie was constantly telling Mary to stop looking at the past, which left Mary with a feeling that she was the obstacle. Ellie wants to move forward while Mary still needs to have her feelings acknowledged. There is an apparent difference in the speed that Ellie and Mary can individually deal with what has happened. Mary is simply not able to think about forgiveness as long as her feelings of anger and sadness are not acknowledged.

We each require varying amounts of time to deal with issues, and this fact becomes one of the greatest stumbling blocks in rebuilding relationships after cheating has occurred. Many times, the one who has cheated has a tendency to look forward to the future, while at the same time the one who has been cheated on needs more time to deal with his or her pain. Acknowledging that we have indeed inflicted pain or that we have been hurt is a crucial part of healing. One very effective way to acknowledge the other person is to see things from his or her point of view, to see the world through his or her eyes.

During the next session, we created space for Mary's feelings through the "See It Through My Eyes" exercise. First Mary had 15 minutes to tell Ellie everything that is upsetting her, what is difficult for her, how she feels and what she would like to change. Ellie's task during this time was to listen, not interrupt and above all to try to fully immerse herself into Mary's vantage point. To do this, Ellie needed to put her own thoughts to one side. When Mary had said all she needed to say, they exchanged places and Ellie sat in Mary's chair. Ellie imagined that she was Mary and told the story again, as if Ellie was Mary speaking. Ellie used "I" statements to do this. Mary listened carefully to find out if Ellie was getting the essentials of her story correctly. This exercise helped Mary to learn how to speak honestly and openly, and Ellie learned active listening skills. When Mary heard her own words from Ellie's voice, Mary felt acknowledged. This was a crucial step for her, and once this had happened, Mary felt ready to look at what their next steps might be. The exercise helped Ellie to understand that she had been moving too quickly, and she felt herself softening as she understood Mary better. Ellie realized that she needed to have more patience with Mary.

Acknowledgement and compassion

Many people find the "See It Through My Eyes" exercise an uncomfortable and strange thing to do. Still, it is an important communication exercise. In particular, the reflection part of the exercise allows the person who has told their story to verify that her or his partner has heard everything, and allows the opportunity to rectify any mistakes or omissions. It often happens that the most important thing that someone has said is the very thing that the other person has not heard or acknowledged. The exercise can also help to clarify differences in nuances between two people. For instance, one person can express a wish that is interpreted by the other person as a demand or requirement.

The exercise also helps develop self-compassion, which is a crucial element when it comes to being able to forgive. When we forgive ourselves and have compassion for ourselves, we can also understand that we are capable of making mistakes. Sometimes the mistakes we make are painful and we need to go through a grieving process as a result. Ellie blames herself for not being honest and that she has hurt Mary deeply. It helps then if Ellie can view herself compassionately. The exercise also helps us to develop the ability to more easily feel compassion for others. Sometimes we blame others because we think that we would never do such a thing ourselves.

For instance, Mary might think that had she been in Ellie's place, she would have made other choices. When she does this she is operating from the premise that Ellie understands, thinks and feels the same way that Mary does. But that is simply not the case. Everyone is unique and thinks, acts and feels differently. We all have different characters based on our unique combinations of qualities, capabilities and blind spots. These sorts of misunderstandings happen all the time. We often take our own points of view as the starting points in our contacts with other people and under-acknowledge differences in personalities. The "See It Through My Eyes" exercise can provoke us to see things through our partners' views and, as a result, to develop compassion.

A FORGIVENESS AFFIRMATION

I forgive you for not being as I am
I forgive you for not living up to my ideal picture
I forgive you for not being perfect.

I forgive myself for the expectations I have
For you, for me, for our relationship
I forgive me for not being perfect.

I forgive you
I forgive me
I release everything.

Revenge and getting even

Often, when we have been deceived or hurt, we have a desire to get back at someone. We want the other person to feel the pain that we feel. In some way, we want there to be an equalizing. Consider the term "get even." If we are hurting, then we want the other person to hurt as well. This need for justice can create feelings of revenge. We all come up with different ways to get even whether we know it or not.

In the following session with Ellie and Mary, we talked about revenge and getting even. What part did this play in their relationship? Mary observed that she wasn't only wounded because Ellie had cheated on her, but she was also hurt because Ellie didn't seem sad. Ellie seemed to be having an easier time dealing with the situation. Mary found herself walking around with a knot in her stomach, with tears in her eyes and intense feelings of sadness and sorrow. Ellie was happy enough to talk about things, and she didn't cry. She was positive and talked of how they could work through it, if they would only look to the future. Mary feels that she takes the relationship much more seriously than Ellie does. Wouldn't Ellie be more upset than she is if she was worrying about the relationship? As a result of her internal dialogue and perceptions, Mary has started to withdraw from Ellie. When Ellie tries to hug her, Mary turns away. In bed, Mary turns her back to Ellie. Mary has started neglecting the house and is not tidying up Ellie's things any more, as if she doesn't care about her. In countless small ways, Mary is inadvertently trying to get even and to eke revenge for her pain.

When I asked Mary what her behavior has achieved, she replied that it has not made her any happier at all. She understood, once she had described it, that she was only driving Ellie away. Ellie noticed that her response to Mary's behavior was to slowly go numb and to not really care anymore; and at the same time, she felt a creeping sense of desperation. She had a feeling that there was nothing more she could do and she had no idea how to tackle it. Instead, she would simply leave the house to escape the unpleasantries. This left Mary feeling even more abandoned.

Revenge and getting even do not, no matter how understandable, contribute to real solutions. They simply drive people apart. The short-term satisfaction may feel good, but it ultimately only creates more stress. Before they know it people who are driven by revenge are stuck in negative circles. It is ineffective to continue an internal dialogue based on negative thoughts about what is happening. Our negative thoughts can affect our health as continuous negativity stimulates our brains and triggers the production of the stress hormone, cortisol. If this occurs over a longer time, we can develop symptoms such as irritability, depression, overemotional behavior, sleep disturbance, bitterness, chronic anxiety and cynicism. That's why it's important to learn to express, and then release, our negative emotions and to become conscious of our desires for revenge and the behaviors that getting even triggers. A better strategy is to talk about our feelings of sadness and anger. It also helps if our partners acknowledge our feelings as often as is required, even if this involves what may seem to be unnecessary repetition.

There are various ways to express our negative emotions and not all are verbal. For instance, it can be helpful to simply write down what we are feeling. Or, some of us find that physical expression such as hitting a punching bag, running, or some other sort of movement can help. Once we do this we can then use our released energy in positive ways, and break negative-behavior circles.

In a new session, I asked Ellie and Mary to carry out an exercise at home. The instructions involved taking ten minutes every day to express themselves to each other. During this time they were not to enter into debates with each other — they were only to listen actively. Their goals were to fully understand where the other person was coming from and to learn to express themselves openly and positively.

In the follow-up session, they explained that this was not an easy task for either of them. It was apparently quite difficult to unlearn their old behaviors and they kept falling back into their habitual discussion mode. So, we repeated the "See It Through My Eyes" exercise. This time it was Ellie's turn. With a third party present, Ellie found her ability to speak freely and openly. She allowed herself to talk about needs that she had kept hidden from Mary until this point — like her need to have an active and satisfying sex life. It became clear that sex is an important part of her persona, and important for her relationship. She didn't want to pretend that this was not the case any more. Ellie also spoke of how important Anne was for Ellie's personal development. This had nothing to do with Mary, it was simply because Anne is different. Ellie thinks Mary is perfectly fine and loves her for who she is. She doesn't want Mary to change at all. Yet, Ellie has a need to grow and to develop other sides of herself that Anne has reawakened.

It was difficult for Mary to reflect back to Ellie what she had heard as she really struggled to see things from Ellie's point of view. It felt very strange to speak of Ellie's needs as if they were her own. She began to increasingly understand how dissimilar they are. Although Mary had always known that she was different from Ellie, she had been unmindful, to some extent, of Ellie's true identity. All of a sudden a more authentic Ellie became clearer to Mary, and Mary understood that Ellie seeks further self-development. This scares Mary as she has no idea what the consequences for their relationship will be. Over the years, Mary had focused more on the partnership and the family they created, and wanted to do as much as possible together. In that way, Mary felt strong and connected. When we started to look at Ellie and Mary's relationship in depth, many signs of codependency appeared.

Codependent relationships

In a codependent relationship, both partners grow into each other to such an extent that we can almost talk of a single unit. Often there is one dominant and one subservient partner. The dominant partner cannot live without the dependence and love of the subservient partner. The subservient partner in turn leans on the dominant partner and enjoys not having to make any decisions or take risks. The basis of the codependent relationship is that each partner looks to the other for what they are lacking themselves, and this creates a feeling of safety. However by doing this, they each end up intellectually and emotionally stunted. In addition, neither partner is truly independent and autonomous, as their own personal identities are pushed to the side. Codependent relationships always come at the expense of one or both partners.

Many women have strong desires for bonding, intimacy and a sense of soul connection. In female-only relationships, needs are often met easily since both partners can have similar desires. Many women tend to focus on relationships and intimacy. Taking care of each other and being involved in each other's lives are important aspects of these relationships. And, there's the pitfall: there is a great chance that the individuality of each partner disappears, that boundaries become less clear and that the two partners are bound to each other through a feeling of happiness. As they spend more and more time together, the partners become increasingly glued to each other. The need for intensity and bonding suppresses autonomy, self-direction and independence.

It is unrealistic to expect that our partners will meet all our needs and desires. If we try to cling too closely to our partners or to our relationships, we will ultimately cease to move. In truly sustainable relationships, partners give each other enough space to continue to develop as individuals. That way, we can continue to choose, as autonomous individuals, to stay with each other in healthy relationships. Free will is always more powerful, and more creative, than rote patterns.

The law of elasticity

In every relationship there needs to be a healthy element of tension, of elasticity. If the first partner takes a bit of a distance from the second partner the tension in the band between them increases and the second partner will have a tendency to move closer to the first one. On the other hand, if the first partner comes too close to the second one then the tension is lost and the second partner will move away to restore it. These kinds of movements happen all the time in healthy relationships. Both partners can do this easily when they have a well-developed sense of autonomy.

When we are autonomous we decide what is good for us. We take responsibility for our actions and we dare to make important choices. We are not dependent on the reactions of the people around us. We're prepared to accept the risks that are inherent in the choices we make. We have a desire to be in charge of our own lives.

In healthy relationships, autonomy and connection balance each other. Autonomy does not mean that we simply do whatever we feel like doing. Instead, we make choices together based on what is good for us and what is good for our partners, families, surroundings, etc. In other words, we balance what is good for others with our own needs for autonomy. When we have a good, balanced sense of personal autonomy — and we know how to maintain and display our own identities — we are often much more attractive to our partners. This attractiveness can in turn increase our partners' desires to be with us; and the passion in our relationships often grows.

Ellie recognizes that in her relationship with Mary, she is often the one that backs away and creates distance from Mary. Mary sees, in her turn, that she is the one who often tries to come closer to Ellie. On the sexual front, however, the dynamic is just the opposite. Mary very often has no interest in making love, and Ellie is the one who mostly takes the initiative. In the meantime, Ellie has discovered that her sexual relationship with Anne is a real source of positive energy and she feels much better about herself as a result.

Mary acknowledges and understands this but the thought of Ellie and Anne making love is too dreadful for her to bear. Yet, Mary knows her own need for sexual contact is much less than Ellie's. The reality is that it was always so, but in the last years it's diminished even more. Mary also admits that she is very concerned about what her lesbian friends will say if they find out what is happening between Ellie and Anne. Their lesbian community is tight, yet Mary does not want to discuss what is going on with her friends, it's all too confusing for her.

If you did what you did,
you got what you got.
—*DUTCH EXPRESSION*

The questions then, for both Ellie and Mary, are: "What can I do differently?" And, "What do I want to take responsibility for?" I asked both of them to make a list of their needs. They then went through their lists, point by point, and explained how they could personally ensure that each need would be met and how the other might help. Mary explained that she needs more time for herself to find out what is important for her. Practically, this means that it would make a big difference if Ellie could come home earlier in the evenings to take care of the children. Mary also said that she would like to know more about what Ellie thinks about, so that she might understand her better. They agreed to set aside 10 minutes every day for Ellie to speak about her feelings and what is important for her.

Ellie, for her part, said that she desired more than simply cuddling with Mary. They made a mutual agreement that they would both take the initiative when it came to sexual contact and that Mary would try to be less reticent. Ellie also said that she would like to re-establish her contact with Anne — more than just the telephone and e-mail level as it was at the moment. Mary said that she was prepared to accept this, but that she found it very difficult. They finally arrived at an interim solution. For the following three months, Ellie would see Anne again, but would not tell Mary where and when they had sex together. In fact, this would be exactly the same situation as when Ellie was cheating, but this time it would be with Mary's tacit approval. During this period Mary and Ellie would both work on enhancing their self-confidence and abilities to be more autonomous. They decided to review their agreement after three months. They would talk about their desires and wishes for the future, and make new agreements as to what form their relationship would take.

Finding our own ways

Every person, and every relationship, is unique. The solutions that work for some people, and the ones that don't, are always surprising. For some, a situation where one partner is pursuing a relationship with someone else but keeping it secret will never work because they feel too attuned to each other, and nothing would be secret. For others, the need for openness and honesty is far too important and it would simply not feel right to ignore important issues. For Ellie and Mary, however, the three month "go ahead, but don't tell me about it" agreement constitutes a temporary solution that brings a level of peace back into their lives. It is an attempt to grow, and a real sign of love on Mary's part to offer this arrangement.

The rewards can be immense when we dare to accept the challenges to explore and discover what works for our unique relationships. If one solution doesn't work out, then we have only come closer to a viable solution as we've eliminated one possibility. We're richer from our experiences and we know ourselves that much better. Most importantly, we can rebuild trust as long as we stay in contact with our partners, talk to each other and keep our agreements with each other.

THE RISE OF THE EGALITARIAN RELATIONSHIP

For thousands of years, personal intimate relationships and marriages have been defined by cultural and social norms. In the overwhelming majority of societies, no matter where in the world they were or are located, the norms have been patriarchal, hierarchical relationships. In other words, there is a clearly defined power and economic structure to marriage, and men were the ones in charge. This has been the case in both monogamous and polygamous marriages and for the most part this state of affairs continues right until the present. However, change is occurring, and it is unstoppable.

The anthropologist, Helen Fisher, author of *Why We Love: The Nature and Chemistry of Romantic Love*, has identified two major trends that are driving this change in relationships: the increasing independence of women, and the fact that people are living much longer. More and more women, especially those in Europe and North America, are discovering that they are no longer dependent on men for their economic security. At the same time, many women are reexamining their lives. They are discovering that defining themselves purely as a mother-caregiver or with a career title is far too limiting.

Simultaneously, an increasing number of men are rejecting the stereotypical role of macho breadwinner and are exploring new, more fully-faceted ways of being. Both men and women are discovering that traditional hierarchical relationships simply do not meet their needs. These trends are important factors in the skyrocketing divorce rates for couples in their forties.

As a result, many people are exploring new and conscious forms of nonhierarchical relationships. Instead of simply trying to conform to roles that have been defined by society, people are looking to create relationships based on good communication, clear agreements and, above all, a recognition that each person in a relationship is equal. These egalitarian relationships have an underlying value: people have equal rights, and all partners have legitimate needs for development and personal expression. If these needs are not met in a healthy fashion, then eventually a relationship will find itself in difficulty.

For many couples, the development of egalitarian relationships encourages awarenesses that some individual needs cannot be met completely within the confines of monogamous relationships. As a result, these couples are consciously exploring alternatives such as open relationships. An open relationship is a relationship where each partner has the option of exploring and maintaining connections with other people with the knowledge and agreement of their partners. These connections can be short or long term, sexual or platonic. The most important point in these egalitarian relationships is that all partners fully acknowledge the rights and needs of each other and are committed to finding ways to encourage each other to fully grow and express themselves. This exploration can, if done consciously and with awareness, allow relationships to deepen and to mature.

Questions you can ask yourself from time to time

+ How do I deal with falling in love?
+ What do I need to be able to forgive?
+ How do I acknowledge my partner for who he or she is?
+ How do I have compassion for my partner and for myself?
+ How do I make space for myself and keep my identity?
+ How do I support my partner's individuality?

Tips for developing autonomy

+ Take a look at your own wishes, boundaries, desires and what drives you. Dare to make space for yourself.
+ Find out what is important for you and why. Look at your values and norms: what are your opinions based on?
+ Take action and do what you enjoy. If you don't know what you enjoy, think back to your childhood: what did you enjoy doing then? How could you do that now?
+ Differentiate between thoughts and feelings. You have feelings, but you are not your feelings. Learn how to manage your feelings instead of letting them manage you. Don't identify yourself with feelings.
+ Transform obstructive and/or restrictive thoughts into positive affirmations and supportive thoughts. Make a list of supportive thoughts that can help spur you into action. For example, "I'm not good enough" can become: "I'm just fine the way I am in this phase of my life."
+ Develop self-compassion: learn how to view yourself in a gentle, respectful and loving way. You're allowed to be different. View yourself with compassion and let go of the temptation to see yourself as a victim.

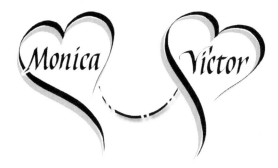

5

Love in the Workplace — Monica

You're happily single and you've got an excellent working relationship with a colleague. You value and respect each other and have accomplished a great deal together. You often bounce around new ideas, and you share the same sense of humor. One day you find yourself in a situation where you call on your colleague for assistance in a personal matter. As a result, your relationship gradually changes and you begin to develop a deeper fondness and affection for each other. But, your colleague is married and you know that a relationship is not on the cards. Still, there is no denying it: you have feelings for each other. What do you do now?

Monica asks herself this question too.

Monica, forty-four, works in a hospital as head nurse in the operating room. She's been divorced for about eight years now, and life as a single woman suits her. Monica is an energetic and autonomous woman who savors her independence and the freedom to make her own choices. She loves her work and enjoys being at the hospital. Her colleague Victor, fifty-one, is a world-renowned neurosurgeon who has earned considerable esteem in the world of medicine. He's been married to Antonia for twenty-three years and they have three children — two teenage boys and an eight-year-old daughter.

Monica and Victor have a good working relationship and they spend a lot of time together at the hospital. Victor is a friendly, attentive and trustworthy man. He is full of integrity, he communicates well and he always takes time to listen to his patients. Monica really likes Victor. They get on very well intellectually and this was of great use recently when a major reorganization took place at the hospital. They shared ideas with each other, and as a result came up with a number of excellent solutions to some challenging problems that had cropped up.

Monica admires Victor and wishes that all the doctors she works with would be like him. She finds him very attractive with his clear blue eyes and his powerful and sensitive hands; and secretly, she's harbored erotic fantasies about him. Monica has always wanted to keep her relationship with Victor purely professional though, and she certainly would not want to land either of them in a sticky situation. She knows that an affair would certainly create problems and difficulties. She has seen close-up the drama that occurred when a nurse she knew had an affair with a married doctor. The nurse in question had ultimately been forced to resign. So, Monica has kept her feelings to herself. At work, Victor was merely a colleague and that was that, until the day Monica's mother fell ill.

After a number of tests, it appeared that the prognosis was not good at all for Monica's mother. Monica's mother lives about an hour from her and the tests were done at a local hospital. The initial results indicated that her mother had a brain tumor. Monica had a feeling that the indicated treatment was not the best one, and she spoke about it to Victor who, as always, was ready to listen. After Monica explained what she knew about her mother's test results, Victor offered to provide a second opinion. Monica was unsure as this would involve considerable traveling for her mother, but at the end of the day her trust in Victor overrode her internal objections. She persuaded her mother to come and see Victor. It turned out that Victor was not at all happy with the suggested course of action from the other hospital, and he offered an alternative, albeit riskier, operation that he would perform himself. After much discussion, Monica and her mother agreed to the new plan.

It was a difficult time filled with tension and worry. Monica was very happy to be able to share her concerns with Victor, even if it she didn't always manage to keep her emotions under control. Their relationship began to gradually take on another character as a result of Victor's intellectual and emotional support, and Monica's need. Victor began to notice that he was thinking more and more about Monica and he felt a desire to be near her. As a professional, however, he focused on the surgery, which, to everyone's relief, was very successful. When the results of the operation were analyzed it turned out that Victor's diagnosis and recommended treatment had indeed been correct. Monica understood that she had Victor to thank for the fact that her mother was still alive. She didn't even want to think about what would have happened if her mother had been treated at her local hospital. She was so happy and relieved! She suggested that it would be wonderful if they could celebrate the successful outcome and floated the idea of a meal for just the two of them at a well-reviewed local restaurant. After a moment of hesitation, Victor agreed.

Three weeks later, it was time for their celebratory dinner. Monica paid extra attention to look just right and put on one of her most attractive, low-cut dresses. Instinctively, she knew that this was a unique opportunity to spend time with Victor in a nonprofessional setting. When Monica arrived at the restaurant, Victor was waiting for her. For the first time, Victor saw Monica in a stunning evening dress, and he was confronted with how attractive she was to him. He could not keep his feelings to himself, and he blushed when he caught sight of her cleavage. This did not escape Monica's attention. In an instant, she realized that the attraction was mutual, and she was thrown into confusion. She never would have imagined it! He always spoke so lovingly about his wife and family. Could he really be interested in her? As they sat at the table together over a lovely meal she could feel the sparks flying between them. It was an incredible evening. They discovered that they are both great fans of opera and classical music, something they hadn't discussed before. Victor stepped into uncharted territory when he asked her about her love life and started to tease her. It almost seemed like he couldn't keep his feelings in check. Monica felt herself responding. She also became aware of the fact that she had a certain power that she could use. It was fascinating that she could bring an otherwise ever-so-composed man into such turmoil. She felt totally comfortable in her power and her femininity. The tension continued to rise between them for the rest of the evening and they instinctively kissed when they said good-bye to each other. And then, the shock of what had just happened hit both of them, and they made their farewells somewhat awkwardly.

Over the next few days, Monica noticed Victor avoiding her. He didn't even poke his head around her office door for a quick chat like he always used to. She guessed that he was feeling guilty for what had happened. A few weeks later, they bumped into each other in the staff room. Victor tried to simply walk away, but Monica grabbed his jacket and pulled him back. She asked him what was going on. She told him that she had really enjoyed their evening together, but that as far as she was concerned they were still colleagues and she missed the friendly contact they had always enjoyed. Victor responded by making it clear that she should expect nothing from him. He did not want to lose his family and he certainly was not interested in an affair. When he said this they were both relieved, and Victor stopped avoiding her.

All was not as before, though. When nobody was watching, Victor would flirt with Monica. Their looks spoke volumes. In public situations, he returned to his professional demeanor. Occasionally, Victor would privately challenge Monica by asking her if she had dreamed about him the previous night, and then confess that he'd been thinking about her all night as well. He would then lightly brush her forehead with his lips, leaving Monica rather confused and bewildered. Once, he told her how he dreamed that she was wearing her evening dress, only this time the dress slipped off.... When their colleagues were present, Victor returned to his reserved and professional behavior. On the one hand, Monica enjoyed all of this. She enjoyed their friendship, and their occasional flirtatious behavior, and she was glad that they had reestablished contact. On the other hand, Monica was disappointed because Victor continued to make it clear that nothing was going to come of it. His family came first now, and always would. Monica was increasingly caught between these conflicting emotions. It was time that someone helped sort this all out — someone who didn't know her, or Victor, and could take a neutral view of the situation. She made an appointment with Leonie.

When relationships change

Most of us are familiar with the phenomenon of love at first sight. In a single second we know: this is different. We may also be familiar with the situation where love develops gradually between two people. We may know, for instance, that a friendship or work relationship can change as the result of some sort of major event in our lives. Sharing important emotions or thoughts with someone can create a kind of intimacy. Suddenly, we discover that the familiar sight of our friends or colleagues touches us in a different way. It's almost like waves of love flow inside us. It's confusing, and we can become oversensitive to our reactions when the other person is near. We feel excitement that we've never noticed before. Once we've headed down this new path, it often feels like there is no turning back. Love is flowing and there is no way to stop it. This is exactly what Victor discovered in his interaction with Monica. Monica, however, had been aware of her attraction to Victor.

What do we do with these changed feelings? Do we dare to acknowledge them? Are they allowed? Some of us can manage them easier than others.

If we acknowledge how we feel for someone else then, eventually, we have to deal with these feelings. It's no longer possible to repress them or rationalize them away, no matter how attractive that option might be. The question soon arises: What do these feelings mean for me? How do they affect my life? What about my partner's life and family? What about my existing relationship? The answers that we give to these questions depend on a number of factors:

- our characters
- choices we've made and things we've experienced earlier in life
- whether we self-identify as polyamorous or not
- if we are open to (complementary) relationships
- whether we are supported by our close friends and families
- the culture we live in and its influence on us
- the norms of the society we live in
- our own personal values and norms
- the values and norms of the person we love
- the values and norms of this person's partner(s)
- the short and the long-term consequences for all parties concerned

All of these factors influence our decision-making processes. Will we, can we, or dare we be open about our feelings? Can we keep our lives balanced without everything falling apart?

When Monica came to see me, I saw a strong and powerful woman; but I also saw a confused person with strong emotions. As she talked about Victor, her gestures became bigger and more animated and as she spoke she became visibly flushed. The situation was clearly very uncomfortable for her. I asked Monica what she felt. She didn't know anymore. She was confused as her otherwise well-ordered life had been turned inside out by the changed relationship to Victor. She told me that she did not ever want to do anything to endanger his marriage or family. Although she enjoyed the additional attention from Victor, she did not want to exploit the situation for her own ends by flirting with him. She respects him as a physician and as a person and views him, just as importantly, as another woman's husband and a father.

I asked Monica what she thought of the fact that Victor flirted with her sometimes. A passionate and dreamy look appeared in her eyes. She admitted that she really enjoyed it. It was wonderful to feel that she could affect him so strongly. On the other hand, she couldn't stand it. It made everything so complicated. "I really should be furious with him!" she shouted. "Are you furious?" I asked.

I encouraged Monica to bring herself to a place of inner quiet and then focus her attention on her feelings when she thought of Victor flirting with her. What did she feel in her body, and where? Monica pointed to her belly, her chest and her throat. She felt surprised, happy, angry, irritated, frustrated, powerless and sad. It was a hodgepodge of both positive and negative emotions. It was no wonder Monica felt confused and that she had no idea what to do! When I asked her what upset her the most, she said: "the contradiction between my feelings of having power and at the same time being powerless."

No one can make you feel inferior
without your consent.
—ELEANOR ROOSEVELT

Power and dependency

We can only have power over another in a relationship if the other person gives us this power and allows us to exercise it. Power and dependency are therefore inextricably connected. If one person leads and the other one automatically follows, then the leader has been given power by the follower, and the follower has assumed a position of dependency. As a result, the follower can be left with a feeling of powerlessness. If we follow simply because it seems self-evident and not as a result of conscious choice, or if we are always adapting to someone else's wishes and boundaries, we hand over our power, and we are indeed powerless. Even more: there is a danger of losing awareness of our own boundaries as we allow the other person's definitions to take precedence over ours. Monica is grappling with this phenomenon.

Power is temporary
and is something others give you,
Strength is infinite and comes from yourself.
—MARIJKE LINGSMA

Monica felt that she had power when Victor flirted with her or when he revealed his attraction to her. He was the one with a relationship and a family. She was single and therefore also free to decide whether to respond to his advances, and this made her feel like she had the upper hand. This quickly changed into a feeling of powerlessness when Victor told her that he was not interested in pursuing a relationship with her and subsequently distanced himself. A feeling of powerlessness occurs when we feel that we have few or no options available and there is nothing left to do but operate within someone else's boundaries.

In her previous professional relationship with Victor, Monica knew exactly where her boundaries were: she had private fantasies concerning Victor but she kept them to herself. Her job and her professionalism were too important for her to do otherwise, and she did not want to interfere in someone else's marriage. To do that would misalign her own personal values and norms, and compromise her sense of integrity. This all changed the moment the attraction between them strengthened.

Although Monica absolutely did not want to have a relationship with a married man, she found herself responding to his flirting. Suddenly she no longer knew what to do with her feelings for him and she was unsure where the boundaries were in this changed relationship. She let herself be led by Victor: he decides what — or what not — to do. She enjoys his flirty moods and she likes the fact that she can knock him a bit off balance. However, when Victor withdraws and keeps to himself — dons his more formal persona — Monica feels rejected, and uncertain. What does Victor really want? What does Monica want? She'd love to simply give into her feelings of wanting to seduce him but that goes against her entire being. Her head is telling her clearly: This man is not for you. He is choosing to be with his wife and family. So what now?

I challenged Monica to play devil's advocate using a technique called "provocative coaching." This is a method that first creates a bit of chaos that later can be distilled into clarity. I laid out a number of imaginary scenarios with exaggerated situations and outcomes. This was all done from a space of love, empathy and complete attention from my side. I told her it is simple. All she has to do is seduce Victor and spend a whole night with him. Then he would understand what she really means to him. Ultimately the love between them is so strong that the best thing they can do is simply enjoy it and throw themselves into it wholeheartedly. She needs to do this properly with some really sexy lingerie, and make sure that he is completely smitten with her on that first night. The only problem is: how to get him into the right place to carry out this plan? She'd have to come up with some creative way of doing this. Maybe she could trick him into meeting her in a hotel room and handcuff him to the bed? There are private detectives you can hire to follow unfaithful spouses — maybe she could hire a few to kidnap him? All Victor would need is one night with her and he would understand how fantastic she is to be with. He would never want to lose her after that and she could be his lover forever. So many other women carry on this way, why not her? All that moral nonsense just makes life dull anyway. Being the lover of a famous neurosurgeon, someone who is world-renowned, that would be great, wouldn't it? OK, she couldn't take him to parties and she would still spend holidays alone, but having a lover who is a top neurosurgeon has one real advantage to it: he has money. Lots of money. If she plays it right she could always wash away her guilt by letting him pay for her to go spend a day or two at a luxury spa. Then she'd be far away, safe from him and his family and in the meantime she could relax and enjoy the Jacuzzi, massages and facials. I continued to fantasize a bit and even more possibilities became apparent. When Monica started to protest I immediately switched to a different scenario.

She was right. It's a ridiculous idea. I suggested that it would be naturally far more logical that Victor would decide that the best thing is that she should disappear from his life. After all she is a threat to him as a powerful man with status, someone whose career is the most important thing next to his wonderful, loving and supportive wife and his family. Maybe he could arrange a lucrative redundancy package for her, which would set her up nicely so that she could move somewhere else and start a new job. That of course would give her ample opportunities for a new career. How long had she worked at the hospital? Twenty years? Much too long actually. Besides, she would get over him soon enough and she was sure to find someone else more suitable. A man who is free and who can be totally there for her. Anyway, it would be just fine if Victor suffered a bit when she was gone. He was the one who started it after all, flirting and teasing her. He should pay for that. Shouldn't he?

As the conversation progressed Monica found herself thrown back and forth between the different scenarios and didn't have much of a chance to escape. This elicited a state of inner turmoil. She felt even more like she didn't know what to do. She didn't want him to disappear out of her life, and she absolutely didn't want to be his lover even if he got down on his knees and begged her. Later on when she went home, she finally realized what she really wants from Victor; to be treated with respect by him — just like she respects him and his boundaries. She doesn't want him to flirt with her anymore and she wants to end the mixed messages. It's time to have an equal relationship with him. Out of the chaos of provocative coaching emerged the space for Monica to get in touch with her role in the situation.

INNER KNOWING

Provocative coaching uses a method that bears some resemblance to a Zen Buddhist koan. A koan is a paradox or a riddle that has no apparent solution and is used to show the inadequacy of logical reasoning.

Two monks were arguing about the temple flag waving in the wind.

One said, "The flag moves."
The other said, "The wind moves."
They argued back and forth but could not agree.

Hui-neng, the sixth patriarch, said:

"Gentlemen!
It is not the flag that moves.
It is not the wind that moves.
It is your mind that moves."

The two monks were struck with awe.

The purpose of a koan is to bring the Zen student into a state of confusion to transcend logical thinking and thereby move forward on the path to enlightenment: a state of judgement-free continuous perception.

Provocative Coaching uses exploration — and ultimately rejection — of opposing scenarios to allow movement beyond reasoning to find a solution that comes from deep within. The Chinese call this inner space of knowing the "second brain" or *dan tian*. In the West, we often refer to it as a "gut feeling" or intuition.

Recent research at the Max Planck Institute for Human Cognitive and Brain Sciences in Munich has validated this age-old concept of a second brain. It appears that there is indeed a vast network of nerves arranged in a complex web in the tissue surrounding our intestines that does act as another center of information processing in our bodies. Professor Wolfgang Prinz hypothesizes that this network is the source for unconscious decisions which the main brain later claims as conscious decisions of its own.

So how does one learn to listen to this second brain? Just think for a second of the sayings we use to encourage calmness and to avoid hasty action: take a deep breath; count to 10; sleep on it. These are all excellent ways to slow down and to allow our inner sense of what is right to surface. However, listening is only the first step. The next step is to trust our feelings, and the final one is to act on them or, at the very least, allow them to be factored in as important and valid input for our decision making processes. It can be scary at first to trust what may seem to be illogical or irrational feelings, but with time you can discover a new source of internal wisdom. Win/win solutions are often the result.

Boundaries and equality

When a relationship changes, so too does its boundaries and definitions. As a result, it can be unclear where the new boundaries are. Who decides what? How do we behave with each other now?

This is the case with Monica and Victor. Although, technically speaking, Victor is her superior, they had developed a working relationship where Monica felt that she was equal to Victor. When her mother was ill, however, this changed. Victor had the skills and experience, and Monica allowed herself to be guided by his expertise. During this time she felt unsure and was quite emotional, and her admiration for Victor's vision, persistence and certainty grew. She ended up putting him on a pedestal and their relationship was no longer equal. This inequality continued as their relationship became more intimate.

Freedom exists in recognizing boundaries.
—KRISHNAMURTI

Freedom and equality

Inequality in a relationship can occur when someone else sets a boundary clearly and we unmindfully accept that boundary as well. On the other hand, equality happens when the choices we make come from our own inner sense of freedom. Then, we are operating from a standpoint of conscious choice. When we make conscious choices, we also choose to accept the consequences of our choices. Freedom is not necessarily free of restrictions or conditions, however. When we act freely, and in a mature fashion, we define our own boundaries and we consider other's boundaries. This is true equality.

Consciously choosing is not always easy as our heads and our hearts do not always agree. When we fall in love with someone who is already in a relationship with someone else there are a number of options we can choose from:

+   Keep our feelings to ourselves and don't say or show anything to our secret love(s).
+   Let our feelings take center stage and try to get our secret love(s) to decide to be with us. We seduce them or start an affair. We let our secret

love(s) deal with their partners and families.

+ We decide to literally leave the situation and not see our secret love(s) any more.

+ We try to find a compromise where we allow our feelings to exist but make clear agreements on how to deal with them, with all the parties concerned, and in a way that everyone finds acceptable.

We can test out each choice by asking ourselves:"Does this choice give me a good feeling or does it simply create more problems? What are the long-term consequences?"

In the following session with Monica, we looked at these different options together. It became quickly apparent that the first three options were not possible in her situation. She had already, for many years in fact, harbored feelings for Victor and she had kept them to herself; but now the situation had changed. Seducing Victor would not work for Monica as it would create new problems and the consequences were unknown and potentially disastrous. The third option was also not a possibility. It would feel terrible to simply exclude Victor from her life. She'd have to find another job and move to another city and she didn't want to do that. So, she carefully considered option number four. This seemed like a solution that fit the situation, but it was also difficult. It felt right to Monica but she also saw problems with it. What did she want? What did such an agreement look like?

Negative feelings as messengers from our needs

If we wish to discover what we truly want (for instance, which option works best) it helps if we can stop and examine the feelings we have for each possibility. Again, in coaching and counseling, there is an understanding that beneath every emotion there is a (sometimes hidden) need. For instance, beneath anger there can be a need for respect and under sadness there can be a need for attention. Every feeling therefore has a message that we can discover when we are open to digging deeper. So when we feel a strong emotion, it can be helpful to simply stop and pay attention and see if we can "listen inside". What is our underlying need? Is there some way to meet this need? What needs require action from the other person?

Monica took a look at her needs by first getting clear about what she was feeling. We then looked at how she might satisfy the needs that were underlying her emotions. To do this we created a schematic diagram to help create a clear overview of her situation

Feeling	Underlying need	How I can meet my need	What I can ask Victor to do
Surprised	To be able to enjoy myself	Do it	
Happy	I want to able to express the joy I feel	If I can't express it to Victor then express it some other way	
Angry	Respect	Discover where my own boundaries lie	Respect my boundaries
Irritated	Peace and clarity	Make a choice	Communicate my choice to Victor and potentially negotiate with him
Frustrated	A need for control	Indicate clearly my boundaries and wishes: stop flirting	
Powerless	A need to decide for myself what I want	Stand up for myself	
Sad	Consolation	Listen to classical music, walk, cuddle with my cat, do fun things with my friends	

Monica found that the most difficult thing for her to do was to find a way to deal with her feelings of love for Victor. She wanted to express the love she felt. Having an affair with Victor was not an option, and Victor had made it clear that there was no chance that his wife would allow him to have a complementary relationship with Monica. Monica didn't see that as a viable solution anyway, even if it had been an option. So, Monica realized if she and Victor were going to continue as friends, they simply had to find another way to express their love for each other. How could they do this if sexual contact was out of the question? Monica took this question home with her to consider. She also made a promise to herself that she would have a conversation with Victor and express her needs to him.

When I saw Monica three weeks later, she was visibly relieved. She had sorted out her feelings and desires. She wanted Victor to stop flirting with her and to stop his on-again and off-again behavior. She wanted to be able to have an ongoing friendship with him, professionally and in their free time. She wanted to be able to enjoy his company outside of work but to keep it at a level of friendship. She also wanted to make space in her life to meet other men and leave open the possibility that she might have an intimate relationship with one of them. She realized that what she wanted was a friendship with Victor, and a friendship that his wife knew about too. She did not want to do anything behind Antonia's back.

Once Monica was clear about all of this, she went and spoke with Victor about it. That conversation had been really good for her. Victor had been completely oblivious to the consequences of his inconsistent behavior towards her. It appeared that he was rather confused due to his strong feelings for Monica and he was quite relieved that she was now setting some boundaries. He told her that he would consider her suggestion that they have a friends-only relationship where they would see each other outside of work once a month and go to a concert or take a long walk together. Victor's wife, Antonia, already knew that Monica is a trusted colleague, and she had heard all about the situation with Monica's mother. What Antonia did not know was the depth of Victor's feelings for Monica. Victor said he needed time to have this discussion with Antonia. First he wanted to sort out the relationship with Monica in the workplace so that it would be easier for them to have a friendship outside the hospital.

Monica felt strong and powerful again after this conversation and she felt like she was back in the driver's seat concerning her life. When I asked her how she decided to deal with her feelings of love for Victor she answered, "The other day, I read about someone else who had dealt with this. The woman had discovered that when she was in love with someone, she also wanted to be loving towards him. For her, being in love was the same as acting lovingly. I recognized myself a bit when I read it. If I feel love for someone, I want to be able to give love. This need of mine is very strong, so I'm going to do what the woman on the forum did. I can be loving towards other people and give them something so that my love can flow. I know it might sound bit silly, but I've decided to visit my elderly aunt a bit more often, and take her out for coffee and on other outings. Does that sound crazy?"

Who decides what is crazy or not? If it works for us and it helps us get to where we want to be, then why not? We decide what works best for us.

Questions you can ask yourself

- If the boundaries I have with someone have been altered, what happened? Who moved the boundary?
- Why has the boundary moved? Is the movement justified? What does this mean for me?
- What feelings recur for me? What do they tell me about my underlying needs?
- Do I dare stand up for my needs? If not, why not? If yes, how do I do it?

Tips for setting boundaries

- Become aware of your emotions and negative feelings. They are messengers from your underlying needs. If you concentrate on your needs it is easier to consider what you really want and therefore it is easier to discover where your boundaries lie.
- Stay true to your own boundaries and personal limits. They are there for a reason. Listen to and respect yourself.
- Indicate your boundaries and express your needs clearly.
- Accept the difficulties that a certain choice can bring with it. By doing this you reclaim your own freedom and you become your own leader.
- Take back your power by expressing what you want irrespective of the outcome or whether it is realistic or not. You can always negotiate afterwards and make another choice.

LOVE UNLIMITED

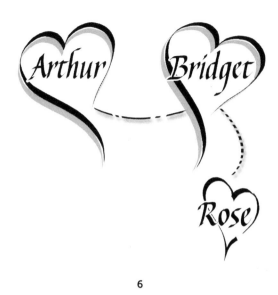

6

A Bisexual Solution —
Bridget, Arthur and Rose

*Y*ou've known for a long time that you are attracted to women. Yet, you are married
to a wonderful man and you have a happy family together. Your feelings for women
have always been there in the background, but you've never done anything with them.
Then, one day you meet a woman who touches you so deeply that you can no longer deny
it. You've arrived at an age, and a point in your life, when you realize that this is an op-
portunity you do not want to miss. You want to explore what it means to make love with a
woman. There's a problem though. Your husband won't go along with it; and if you accept
this woman into your love life, you will break the agreement you made long ago.

Bridget found herself dealing with this dilemma.

Bridget is thirty-eight; and she and Arthur, forty-one, married sixteen years ago.
They have a fifteen-year-old daughter. Bridget works as a civil engineer at a construction company and Arthur is a real estate agent. They'd met each other at work. Arthur
had been impressed by Bridget's dedication to her job and her ability to think and
work quickly. Bridget felt attracted to Arthur's ability to communicate clearly and get
along easily with people. They are good partners all round, including their knack for
sharing and solving work problems together.

Bridget has known from a very early age that she is bisexual. As a teenager she kissed a few girls but it had never gone further than that. She never spoke to anyone about her feelings for girls. Homosexuality, let alone bisexuality, was unmentionable in the small village where she grew up. She had, however, read books on the subject, enough to know that she was indeed bisexual. Both women and men figured in her erotic fantasies. She loved to look at women when she walked around town, and always admired their sensuous poise.

When Bridget first met Arthur, she was head over heels in love with him. Just before they got married she decided that she needed to tell him about her feelings for women. When Bridget finally brought it up, Arthur was a bit surprised. He'd never noticed a thing. He asked her what this would mean for their relationship because, as far as he was concerned, he expected a monogamous relationship and there would be no nonsense with anyone else, not even women. "Of course not," she responded with a laugh. "I'm crazy about you, you know that. I love you, and I don't want to lose you." Arthur appeared to be reassured. "Honey, I love you and I accept that you find women attractive. As long as you don't do anything with anyone then that's fine by me." And that seemed to be the end of the discussion.

With the birth of their daughter, Bridget's feelings for women were totally set to one side as she and Arthur both focused all their attention on their family and careers. There were times, though, when Bridget would be more aware of women and would even have erotic dreams about them. When she awoke after one of these dreams, she would be surprised at herself, but also uncomfortable when she saw Arthur innocently sleeping next to her. She had once nudged Arthur when she noticed a beautiful woman walk by their table at a café, but his irritated reaction ensured that she'd never do that again. So Bridget kept her feelings for women to herself. She did have a couple of lesbian friends that she got along really well with, and these friendships helped her to feel like a whole person.

Things had changed in the last few years however, and Bridget found herself fantasizing about women more and more. Her dreams were full of them. It seemed like there was no way of avoiding her attraction to women anymore and eventually she realized that she was going to have to do something about it. During the last couple of months she started to browse dating sites for women. She was astounded that women dare to put their pictures up on the Internet! She'd never do that herself, but she continued to look....

Bridget works with calculations and computers. It is a very technical job and to some extent she finds herself stuck in her head. A few months ago, she decided to balance this out and attended a Biodanza class. She'd heard positive things about Biodanza from her friends and she was curious. She was attracted even more when she discovered that Biodanza is all about personal growth and learning to make conscious contact with other people and ourselves. She was a bit nervous at the thought of doing something so very different from what she was used to, but it was time for a challenge.

At the first Biodanza evening session, Bridget met and felt immediately drawn to Rose, a friendly and attractive woman. During one of the dances, they gazed into each other's eyes for what seemed like ages and at the end of the dance, hugged each other. At first, Bridget was surprised, but even though they had just met, it felt natural and right to be hugged by Rose. At the end of the evening they found themselves deep in conversation. Rose introduced herself. She is a forty-five-year-old naturopath and has been attending Biodanza for years. She explained that Biodanza, or "healing dance" as she calls it, is very important to her, and she attends as much as she can. Bridget felt that she'd stepped into a new and unknown world, but one that she needed to experience. Later that evening, she spoke enthusiastically with Arthur about her impressions of the dancing and about meeting Rose. Arthur was delighted for her. It was all a bit too "airy-fairy" as far as he was concerned, and it was definitely nothing that he was personally interested in. If it made Bridget happy, though, then he was fine with it and he encouraged her to carry on.

The Biodanza evenings had a significant and positive effect on Bridget's life, and she began to feel closer and closer to Rose. At the end of the dance evenings, they always sat and chatted over tea, and they were often the last people to leave. Bridget noticed that she was definitely attracted to Rose and this confused her. At home she continued to look into how other women dealt with similar situations. She read a number of postings on women-only forums that spoke of how important it is for bisexual women to talk to their partners about what is going on in their lives. How could she talk with Arthur about this? Although Arthur had said that he accepted Rose's bisexual attractions, he always reacted in a way that indicated that he was very uncomfortable whenever she spoke about women.

At the same time, Bridget's bond with Rose was intensifying. Rose revealed that she was bisexual; and she and her husband had an explicit understanding that she could have sexual contact with women. Rose told Bridget that she had been involved in a complementary relationship before. That relationship lasted a few years, until the woman moved away. Rose's lifestyle suited her, and her husband, perfectly.

Bridget was impressed with how easily Rose spoke of the way she had organized her life. Bridget wished that she could create such a situation for herself. As Bridget listened to Rose, her imagination took off. She began to imagine herself kissing and making love to Rose, and Bridget felt her desire to spend time with Rose growing and growing.

On the way home, Bridget thought about what Rose had said and it became clear to her that if she really wanted to spend time with Rose, then there was no way around the fact that she had to talk to Arthur about it. She had a strong sense that if she met up with Rose somewhere other than the Biodanza venue, something would definitely happen between them. So that was that. She decided that she was going to talk to Arthur.

When she arrived home, Arthur was relaxing on the couch sipping a glass of wine. She suddenly hesitated and thought about what this discussion might do to him. She wanted to talk to him, but didn't know how. Instead, she told him that she was tired and she went to bed. Arthur found this very strange. She was usually so enthusiastic and full of life when she came home from Biodanza. He knew her well enough to know that something was up, and he followed her into the bedroom. He sat down on the bed and gently but persistently kept asking her what was happening until she finally admitted it. She told him that she was attracted to Rose and that she wanted to make a date with her. She wanted to find out what it feels like to make love with a woman. She no longer wants to suppress that side of her.

Arthur was shocked. He'd known that Bridget enjoyed meeting and dancing with Rose, but he had not seen this coming at all. Attracted to women? Bisexuality? What on earth is she talking about? Bridget reminded him of the conversation before they were married. Slowly, Arthur began to remember. But that was so long ago! She'd never said a thing to him about her feelings for women during all the years they'd been together. He thought she simply went through some kind of youthful confusion about her sexual identity, but that was long over. Aren't they married to each other? He had always assumed that she, just like he was monogamous. If she wants to explore this she'd better understand that their marriage was no longer on a firm footing.

Arthur was angry and reacted strongly. Bridget, deeply disappointed at his reaction, retreated into herself. For a few days afterwards they avoided each other and barely spoke. Arthur threw himself into his work, and Bridget sat for hours talking with the women through the web forum. They advised her to talk to him, "Explain to him how important it is for you. If you get stuck, try to find some professional help." Bridget thought this was sound advice, so when she found Leonie's web site she called her for an appointment. Leonie suggested that she come with her partner as the situation clearly affected both of them. Bridget talked to Arthur about this and he readily agreed. He had the feeling that his marriage had suddenly been thrown into disarray and getting assistance from a knowledgeable third party seemed like a good idea.

Agreements and expectations

When we fall in love and form relationships we tend to have many unspoken expectations as to how the relationships will unfold and how we will interact with our partners. On top of this, we each have our own perceptions and ideas about sexuality and intimate relationships. The most common unspoken agreement we have is that if we are in a relationship, we will be faithful to each other. Most people assume that if we are in a relationship we will not have sex or engage in intimate acts with anyone other than our partners. In actuality, our boundaries and limits vary.

For some men, being faithful means that they simply do not have any female friends, whereas for others it's the most normal thing in the world to have women as friends. For some people, a cup of coffee with a member of the opposite sex is too much, while for others it's perfectly fine to stay at a friend's house overnight. For some, it's even fine to sleep in the same bed since they know and respect each other's boundaries. For others, that would be completely out of the question as you only share a bed with your partner because "bed equals sex" and they can't imagine that you would share a bed with someone of the opposite sex without having sex. How we think and deal with sexuality in friendships and relationships is different for each one of us and is based on our own (spoken and unspoken) personal values and norms.

Bridget and Arthur had their own personal ideas and visions of sex and relationships when they met, and they had also made an explicit agreement in this area. It was completely clear that extramarital sex was out of the question for both of them. At the time Bridget made the agreement, sex outside her relationship with Arthur hadn't even crossed her mind. She was in love with Arthur and there was no room for another person in her life. She assumed that she was monogamous and whether that involved a man or a woman was not the issue. Of course, it was handy that she had ended up with a man as heterosexuality is much more accepted in our society. It also meant that there would be no unpleasantness with her parents and family, which would certainly have been the case if she had decided to have a long-term relationship with a woman. Heterosexuality was also a simpler solution when it came to starting a family. The result of all of this was that she concealed her bisexuality by marrying Arthur. They presented themselves to the world as a heterosexual couple and she agreed, without further ado, to Arthur's request for a monogamous relationship. What she didn't realize at the time was that her sexual needs could change over time. She could never have imagined the impact that her sexual identity would have on her life several years later.

During our first conversation, it rapidly became clear that Bridget and Arthur had very different perceptions of the agreement they had made and their mutual expectations. Arthur told me that he felt that Bridget had been a bit duplicitous now that she had suddenly decided that she had different sexual desires. For him, Bridget was a normal heterosexual woman that enjoyed having sex with him as a man. He did not understand why she would put her family and relationship at risk by deciding to experiment with a woman. Above all, being faithful is a core issue for him as they had promised each other exclusivity when they married. Was that no longer worth anything to her?

Bridget then explained her side of the story to me. She told me how she had always had feelings for women and that they had never disappeared. However, Arthur's discomfort caused her to keep her feelings to herself. Still, just because she never said anything did not mean that the feelings didn't exist. Just the opposite, they are an important part of who she is. Until now, it had always been an inner experience — she would look at women, enjoy seeing them and even dream and fantasize about them. In general, she had always found the soft, round contours of women's bodies nicer than men's. "What about me then?" interrupted Arthur. "We have sex, don't we? You enjoy it? You're not going to tell me we have a bad sex life are you?" he shouted angrily. Bridget said that she, to the contrary, enjoys their lovemaking and always has. It's just that her attention has been drawn to women lately. She was curious, she told him, to know what it would be like to make love with a woman. She simply wanted to find out. She had a feeling that there was a piece missing in her life, that somehow it wasn't complete. "You're a man, with a man's body. That's wonderful, I wouldn't want it any other way" she told him earnestly. "It's simply that I would like to experience what it is like to be with a woman," she said with tears in her eyes. "I know, I also feel guilty. Am I allowed to ask for this? Why can't I just continue the way I was and have it be enough for me to be with you? If I could simply be heterosexual, we wouldn't be in this mess and we wouldn't be sitting here!"

Bisexual myths

The majority of the population consider themselves heterosexual. Heterosexuality is also the norm in most cultures. However, approximately ten percent of the Dutch population self-identify as either gay or lesbian which corresponds well with the figure of one in ten often cited in the United States. Bisexuals are neither completely homosexual or completely heterosexual. Research in the last years has shown that bisexuality occurs in the brains of all of us. Whether this tendency is developed or not is influenced by the amount of the male sex hormone, androgens, that a child in the womb is exposed to. According to the world-renowned sexologist Alfred Kinsey, there is a large gray area between being one hundred percent homosexual and one hundred percent heterosexual. This gray area is what is commonly referred to as bisexuality. Sexual identity is therefore not the black and white story that some make it out to be. Most of us, however, need clarity in this area and want to know where we stand.

When are we bisexual (bi)? If we have erotic fantasies about both men and women? If we are stimulated when we see two people of the same sex having sex together? Are we only bisexual if we act on our desires physically? Or is it only when we want to have a relationship with a man and a relationship with a woman at the same time? The answer is not so clear.

Myths and misunderstandings concerning bisexuality:

- Bisexuality is simply a transition phase for gays and lesbians
- Bisexuals are, as a result of their sexual identity, not monogamous
- Bisexuals cannot, as a result of their sexual identity, be faithful
- Bisexuals don't dare choose
- Bisexuals are oversexed

Bisexual identity

In 2008, forty-thousand Dutch people filled in a questionnaire called "How Bi Are You?" on the web site http://www.hoebibenjij.nl (hoebibenjij means howbiareyou). Parts of the questionnaire were based on the "Klein Sexual Orientation Grid" developed by Dr. Fritz Klein in 1985 and examined diverse aspects of how we experience sexuality (sexual orientation, sexual fantasy, sexual behavior, emotional preferences, social preferences, hetero/homo lifestyle and self-identification). The questionnaire also examined how people see themselves (heterosexual, bisexual, homosexual, mostly heterosexual or mostly homosexual). One of the most remarkable results showed that one percent of the respondents who consider themselves fully heterosexual also responded that they have sexual contact *exclusively* with members of the same sex! Our self-descriptions, therefore, do not always match up our actual behaviors.

The difference is even greater when we look at our fantasies. Only sixty-seven percent of the male respondents and fifty-three percent of the female respondents consider themselves one hundred percent heterosexual. Twenty-five percent of the men who consider themselves heterosexual fantasize about sex with both sexes and, quite remarkably, forty-six percent of the women who consider themselves heterosexual fantasize about having sex with both men and women. Although the survey in question was not scientific and the respondents were not necessarily representative of society as a whole, it is still evident that bisexuality is a complex issue and that there may be more bisexual people than previously credited.

Society and social environments have a large influence on the development of our sexual identities. The push toward heterosexuality is great and this makes life for some bisexuals difficult. Bisexuals often find it unpleasant to have their sexual identities labeled as such. They struggle with all the myths and assumptions that this label conjures. Why it is necessary to label sexual identity at all? They simply want to do what feels natural, with the agreement of all involved.

Other bisexuals find the term "bisexual" just perfect. It creates clarity and gives them an identity to hold on to. It clarifies more options than simply male and female; male and male; or female and female. It creates space for people to question them. Many bisexuals claim, "I don't fall in love with men or women, I fall in love with people." And then there are people who have always felt attracted to a certain gender and then all of a sudden find themselves in love with someone of the other gender. Or, there are those who feel themselves sexually attracted to both men and women but only feel emotionally attracted to one or the other. Bisexuality exists in all forms and variations. On top of this, our personal experiences of sexuality can change over the years.

Bridget relates to this since she has always considered herself bisexual, but never acted on it. Now, she has a growing need to experience her bisexuality and wants to find out what sex with a woman, and in particular with Rose, is like.

In the following session we explored how Bridget sees herself as a bisexual woman and the different aspects of her sexual identity. We used the "Klein Sexual Orientation Grid" for this and created one with three columns; one for the past, one for the present and one representing Bridget's ideal.

Variable	Past	Present	Ideal
Sexual Attraction	Men and women	Mostly to women	Arthur and a woman
Sexual Behavior	Only with Arthur	Only with Arthur	With Arthur and with a woman
Sexual Fantasies	Men and women, sometimes sex with both	Mostly about women, predominantly about Rose	With Arthur and Rose
Emotional Preference	Arthur and girlfriends	Arthur, girlfriends and Rose	Arthur, girlfriends and Rose
Social Preference	Men and women	Men and women	Men and women
Heterosexual/ Homosexual Lifestyle	Hetero lifestyle, lesbian friends	Hetero lifestyle, lesbian friends	Bi lifestyle, able to be open about my bisexuality
Self Identification	Bisexual but more hetero than lesbian	Bisexual	Bisexual

We then looked at Bridget's grid with Arthur present. How strongly does Bridget feel attracted to women and men? Where does she see herself in her sexual identity? What are her fantasies? What is the difference between her current situation and her ideal picture? As we explored these questions, it became clear for Bridget that she found it difficult to accept the consequences of considering herself bisexual. "If only I had a button that I could push that would make me stop finding women attractive," she sighed. It turned out that she was just as afraid as Arthur was of what might happen if she acted on her desire. What would be the effect on their relationship? Would she be able to deal with it emotionally? How would this affect her sex life with Arthur?

I asked Bridget to rate her desire to have sex with a woman on a scale of one to ten where one equals no desire and ten equals infinitely great. For her it was a nine. That had not always been the case though. Previously, when she had sexual fantasies, she did fantasize about women, but not always. She certainly had not had the desire to do anything about it in real life. Her desire at that time had been maybe a two or a three. In the last few years the desire had grown to seven. The stimulation and excitement that Rose had elicited in Bridget increased her desire to have sex with a woman to a nine or possibly even a ten. Bridget was clear that she had a strong desire to have sex with women, but certainly not with other men. As far as she was concerned there was only one man for her, and that man was Arthur.

Bridget was relieved when she began to get more perspective around her bisexuality. The exercise also helped Arthur to understand that Bridget really is bisexual, even though she had until this point been leading a heterosexual life. That was very difficult for him. He had a feeling that all of a sudden he was no longer good enough, because in his view what he had to offer as a man was no longer enough for Bridget. He did admit, though, that the thought of his wife having sex with another woman was not entirely unpleasant. Still, his fears outweighed any inklings of excitement.

I asked Arthur and Bridget to, over the coming weeks, write down all of their fears and concerns and any thoughts they might have about these fears. We would look at these in a future session. I also asked them to write descriptions about the role sexuality plays in their relationship. In addition, I asked them to create a summary of all the positive aspects of their relationship. What was the connection between them? What made their relationship special? What were they good at doing together?

Positive attention

Many couples struggling with the fact that one of the partners has a desire to experience some form of intimacy outside their relationship have the tendency to focus, above all, on the negative aspects of their relationship. The aspects that are going well seem to disappear quickly into the background. The problems, then, are often experienced as more difficult than is really necessary. It is important to stay aware of the positive aspects of the relationship and particularly those characteristics that make it special and strong. Often, these special qualities and strengths contain the keys to the solutions needed.

During the subsequent session, we talked about what was going well in Bridget and Arthur's relationship. Arthur spoke of his admiration for Bridget's honesty and that he was very happy that she had spoken to him before anything took place with Rose. Arthur and Bridget agreed that they are true friends, and that they are genuinely interested in each other. They are enthusiastic about and support each other's work and careers. They also give each other the space and freedom to do what is important for each one of them individually. For instance, Arthur regularly goes on sailing weekends with his friends. Bridget really appreciates Arthur's thoughtfulness and caring. He is the one who always makes a big breakfast for the whole family on Sunday mornings. When it comes to sexuality, they both agree that it has an important place in their relationship although at the moment it is more important for Bridget than for Arthur.

We then took a look at the most important connections between Arthur and Bridget using *The Relationship Game*. The emotional connection turned out to be the most important aspect for both of them. We also considered which connections would be helpful for them in their current situation. The aspects they chose were Learn From Each Other, Feel Equal To Each Other and Trust Each Other.

One of the sticking points for Arthur was that they had agreed to be faithful to each other. Now Bridget wants to break that agreement. As they discussed this they soon realized "faithful" meant different things to each of them. Bridget feels she is faithful to Arthur. She made it clear to him that years ago she chose a life with him and, as far as she was concerned, nothing had changed in that regard. She couldn't imagine a life without him and their family. She didn't want to imagine it either. He was the most important person in her life. She was not looking for another partnership, she was looking for a way to explore and express her sexual feelings for women. She would like to experience that part of her being. In short: she wants to be faithful to him but she also wants to be faithful to herself.

As we spoke, Bridget acknowledged that she wanted to learn how to express her deeper feelings to Arthur. In turn, Arthur said that he would like to learn how to listen better to Bridget without instantly judging her or injecting his opinion as he was prone to do. With some difficulty, Arthur finally voiced his fear of losing Bridget. He said that his concern that she would leave him was the most prevalent reason for him to stop all the discussion about Bridget and women. He just didn't know how to live with what was happening or how to deal with it in a constructive fashion. He saw that he had tried, over the years, to simply not talk about it, and had hoped that her bisexuality would simply go away. Now that Bridget was speaking so openly and in-depth about her bisexuality, he realized that he could not change her, or himself. At the end of the day he is a man, not a woman. If this was something that was so important for her then maybe he would have to find some way to live with it. He could never compete with a woman. But there was a very clear caveat; a woman might be OK, another man would be out of the question. For Bridget that was easy, and she quickly reassured Arthur that he is the only man for her.

As the ramifications of this began to sink in, Arthur started to ask some questions. Did it have to be with Rose, the woman she saw every week? Couldn't it be with someone who lived a bit further away, not quite so close? Were there no other possibilities? Bridget didn't think so, but admitted that it was worth discussing other options. We held a brainstorming session and looked at all the possibilities that there might be for Bridget to meet her need for sexual experience with a woman. We didn't discuss the ideas that came up, we simply listed as many as possible no matter how crazy or impractical. Arthur and Bridget then took the list home to sift through and discuss the different ideas.

A few weeks later, Arthur and Bridget came back and admitted that the bulk of the suggestions had been discounted immediately. The idea of going to a swingers club was put in the bin right away, Arthur couldn't conceive of them doing such a thing. Bridget was not interested in going to a dance evening for lesbian women either. Above all, it became clear that it is indeed with Rose that Bridget wants to explore her bisexuality. She feels incredibly attracted to Rose, and Bridget is not interested in spending intimate time with just any random woman. For Bridget, it is important to feel a reciprocated attraction to someone she has sex with. Her desire to have a sexual experience with a woman is intimately connected to her friendship with Rose.

Bisexual desires and experiences

Men and women do not always experience sex in the same way, and their (bi)sexual expression can also differ. For some, it is possible to have sex if they have solely an emotional connection with someone, while for others there needs to be physical attraction as well. There are also people who can have sex with just about anyone as long as there is a mutual desire for sexual satisfaction. These people make a clear distinction between love and lust, between sex and emotional connection. Some bisexual men have feelings of lust towards men, but are looking for love and an emotional connection with a woman. They couldn't conceive of a partnership with a man. For many people, sex solely for sex's sake is inconceivable because, for them, sex is inextricably connected to the romance and love of an intimate relationship.

So it's easy to imagine that if we are in a heterosexual relationship and our partner connects love with sex, it can be very difficult to tell our partners of our sexual attraction to someone of the same sex. It's not surprising that many bisexual men fulfill their need for sexual contact with other men through secret meetings. Their sense of excitement and sexual tension is often enhanced by the secrecy involved. Sex for them is a short-term sense of satisfaction. These men are often very concerned about endangering their relationships and so they conceal their desires and bisexual activities from their partners. Other men, however, speak openly with their partners and work together to find ways to create opportunities for bisexual activities. Some couples enjoy going to swingers clubs together. This way they can both be aware of each other's activities and incorporate the bisexuality into their own love life. In yet other cases, the bisexual partners are given permission to simply go out and do what they want and to leave the other partners out of it. The point is that what we choose to do with our sexual relations is not important, rather it is critical to make conscious choices and to be able to be fully responsible for the decisions that we do make. Ultimately, it's our lives, and our relationships. That is why it is so important to dare to expose our desires, and to discover what our partners' boundaries are. If we can speak openly, and have the courage to stretch our boundaries we can often come up with creative and rewarding solutions that satisfy everyone. Good communication skills are essential.

> *Our sexuality is such a core part of our being,*
> *such a fundamental part of our identity,*
> *that a part of ourselves dies so to speak if we consciously*
> *or unconsciously deny or suppress it.*
> — ANNEMARIE POSTMA

Arthur initially did not want to know about Bridget's bisexual feelings. By not taking Bridget seriously when she spoke of her feelings for women, or by simply being unwilling to talk to her about them, he unintentionally tried to force Bridget to behave as if her feelings did not exist. He was longing for the simple and straightforward life they had always enjoyed, and hoped that Bridget would stop talking and thinking about women. For Bridget though, the process was unavoidable and she could no longer suppress her feelings. Arthur knew instinctively that this was indeed the case. His relationship is very important to him and that is why he came along to the relationship coaching. He was really afraid for the future and what might happen to their marriage.

In one of our sessions, we investigated Arthur's worries and fears with the help of a visualization exercise where Arthur imagined a disastrous result to their situation. What was the worst that could happen? By creating an image of his worst-case scenario and filling in the details, Arthur realized that his greatest fear was that Bridget would fall in love with Rose and that they would have such incredible sex that Bridget would realize that Arthur was no longer needed. He was afraid Bridget would leave him. One of the most disturbing thoughts for him was the idea that he — a man — would no longer be enough for his wife. We then looked at what thoughts Arthur could create that would support him rather than disturb him. Arthur came up with "As a man I can offer everything that is required of a man; I'm good just as I am. I fully support Bridget in her explorations and they do not make me any less of a man." We also looked at Arthur's underlying needs and asked how they could be fulfilled. He thought that it might help if Bridget could find a way to give him a bit of extra reassurance that he was still important to her, and that she still found him attractive and desirable. In addition, Arthur expressed a strong need for Bridget to be open and honest about what she is doing so that he would know what is happening and where. So he asked Bridget to keep the lines of communication open. He also asked for clear agreements. He wants to be able to apply the brakes if it all becomes too much for him.

Making clear agreements

The ability to make clear agreements is a very important skill to cultivate if we decide to open up our relationships. It is essential that if we do make agreements, we keep them. When a relationship changes, there is a period of flux, and it can be difficult to maintain our trust for our partners. When we keep agreements, we make it clear that our partners and our relationships are important to us, even when things are not going the way we would like in a given moment. A helpful strategy can be to make agreements for a fixed period, to reevaluate in good time, and to adjust the agreements if required.

It was difficult for Bridget to make such a clear agreement ahead of time. She hadn't even had a date with Rose and they were still exploring their friendship. She did have a strong sense that something could happen between them, but ideally, she wanted to be able to simply let things happen and to be able to respond spontaneously. Since Arthur expressed a need for structures and agreements, Bridget felt obliged to consider limits. They agreed, therefore, that Bridget would not have sex with Rose on the first date. Kissing and cuddling was fine but the clothes needed to stay on. Arthur wanted to find out how that would be for him and how that would be for Bridget. They also agreed that she would come home before midnight and that she would send a text message when she left Rose's house. They agreed further that they would talk again after the first date to decide what to do next. Of course, all of this was dependent on what Rose wanted as well. Arthur found it quite exciting and at the same time a bit nerve-wracking, but he was prepared to try the arrangement.

After the next dance evening, Bridget and Rose decided to go home to Rose's house for a bite to eat. Rose's husband greeted Bridget warmly and then bid them both good night and headed off to bed. The women sat down on the couch in the living room. It soon became apparent that Bridget's hunch was correct, Rose was very attracted to her and Rose made no attempt to conceal the fact. Rose put on some sensuous dance music and pulled Bridget up out of her chair to dance with her. They got totally lost in each other and started kissing without even thinking about it. Bridget felt like she had finally come home. It was different to feel a woman's body and to kiss a woman! It felt one hundred percent right and she felt completely relieved. It was exactly like she thought it might be. She thoroughly enjoyed Rose's female energy and it excited her sexually. Bridget remained completely mindful of her agreement with Arthur, though, and she told Rose about it. When Rose heard about what Bridget and Arthur had agreed, she said that she had no problems at all with it. It was important for her, especially since it was Bridget's first time, that it be a relaxed, fun and happy occasion if they did make love. As far as she was concerned, that could only happen if everybody felt good about it, including Arthur.

Rose told Bridget that she looked forward to a "friends with benefits" type of relationship. For her, that meant that she would be delighted to see Bridget once in a while, with lovemaking as a possibility, but without specific commitments. Bridget was very happy to hear Rose's response. Bridget couldn't believe her luck and she felt like she was flying! That this was possible, that she could do this, in her life! She couldn't wait to share her happiness with Arthur and sent him a text "It was great! I'm so happy! And, I really want you... don't go to bed yet ;-) xxxx." Safely home, she found Arthur waiting for her full of excitement. Bridget was so happy to see him that she threw her arms around him and, before they knew it, they were making love in the living room. Afterwards they sat and chatted and Bridget told him everything that had happened. Arthur was relieved and truly happy for her. He was a bit nervous but he had a good feeling about Rose and the way she was approaching Bridget. She seemed to be a trustworthy person. Bridget was very happy that Arthur reacted so positively. It made it much easier for her to share her feelings with him and she felt like it brought them closer together.

The transition from one partner to another

The way we react when we have sex with someone other than our partners varies. For some of us it can have a positive influence on our sex lives and generate a real boost when we come back home. And, some of us need time to make the transition from one sexual partner to another. If we find ourselves in such situations, it's a good idea to observe carefully how we react and, if necessary, talk to our partners about it.

There is no right or wrong here, each person is different. It probably goes without saying that it's useful to know how we function ourselves, and what our partners can do to meet our needs. In fact, some partners are quite happy if there is a bit of distance. Then they can take some time to get used to the idea that their partners have been intimate with someone else.

In our final session, we took a look at what agreements Arthur and Bridget would like to make and for what length of time. I asked them to both make a list of important points to indicate what their needs were in this new situation. For instance it wasn't just about how often Bridget and Rose would meet, but also about what level of detail Bridget and Arthur would reveal to each other. And what about the rest of the world? What did they want to tell their daughter? After both of them had written down their issues, they exchanged lists and discussed them. Bridget and Rose wanted to see each other every other week in addition to the Biodanza evenings. Arthur found once every six weeks more than enough. He was afraid that their relationship would become too intense otherwise and he felt that he'd been more than accommodating already. On top of that, they both had busy lives, and a daughter who knew nothing of what was happening. Arthur wanted to keep things that way, and preferred that they speak of Rose as a "regular" friend. After some discussion, they finally agreed with each other that Bridget and Rose could see each other once a month. Bridget would not tell Arthur all the details of her time with Rose as she wanted to keep that for herself. They also agreed that except for Bridget's best friend, they would not tell anyone else about it. The agreement would be for six months, and they would revisit it then. They also promised each other to be honest about what they were experiencing and to keep talking to each other, even if things turned out differently than they expected.

Put up in a place
where it's easy to see
the cryptic admonishment
T. T. T.
When you feel how depressingly
slowly you climb,
it's well to remember that
Things Take Time.
— a 'grook' from PIET HEIN

TRADITIONAL CHINESE MEDICINE
AND SUPPRESSED SEXUALITY

Traditional Chinese Medicine (TCM) is the term for the healing system that is used by Acupuncturists, Chinese Herbalists and Tui Na (Chinese Massage) practitioners, among others. It is one of the oldest systems of healing known to man and has been practiced for thousands of years. Underlying TCM is a system of energy observation and awareness that is useful not only for healing physical problems but also emotional ones. A particularly pertinent insight from TCM has to do with treating chronic situations: it can take up to one week of treatment for each year that one has encountered a chronic problem.

Another basic tenet of TCM is that the fundamental cause of disease ("dis-ease") is obstruction and/or blockage in our internal energy matrix. Many of these blockages are caused by rigidity in our systems; and softening our systems to allow this rigidity to melt away is a core methodology employed by TCM.

In many ways, relationships are no different. Entrenched beliefs, fear-based prohibitions and poor communication can all be symptoms of a relationship that has become rigid and therefore may be blocking the flow of energy needed to keep it healthy.

Suppressing sexuality, from an energetic point of view, means blocking or obstructing a particularly powerful element of life energy. The blocking can be both internal (self-denial) and external (lack of expression). To gently move forward based upon communication, trust and love is completely in accord with the TCM idea of becoming less rigid. Taking time is of paramount importance, as this allows the newly-unblocked relationship energies time to adjust, adapt and grow.

Questions to ask yourself

+   How do I communicate with my partner about my sexual desires?
+   How do I view bisexuality? How does this express itself, if at all, in my life?
+   Do I dare to be open about my (bi)sexuality?
+   What erotic fantasies would I like to have come true? Do I dare speak about this to my partner? If so, do I do it? If not, why not?
+   What do any sexual desires that my partner might have mean for our relationship?

Tips for opening your relationship when bisexuality is present

- Accept your partner's bisexuality. Acceptance is more than simply tolerating. Complete acceptance means that you accept your partner for who she or he is and that you do not try to change her or him. It means that you display interest in how each of you sees the world. This also means that you explore how your relationship is affected and that you talk about this with each other.
- Take charge of your sexuality. Explore what (bi)sexuality means for you and talk about this with your partner. One way to do this is to use the Klein Grid Orientation Scheme.
- Be open with each other about your feelings, your expectations, your wishes and your behaviors. Good communication is essential for this. If you discover that you have difficulties communicating, then work on those skills first.
- Take small steps and take time. Make sure that both of you realize what each step means for the other person. Keep talking.
- Have respect for each other's boundaries.
- Understand that when you try something new, it might not work out the way you expected it to. Learn from your experiences and think about how you can use knowledge about what works and what doesn't for future decisions or agreements.
- Keep each other informed as to how the development of your bisexual experiences are progressing and decide how much detail you want to tell each other. What is private for you and what do you want to share with your partner? What do you, as a partner, want to know? What are the benefits of knowing?
- When making changes in your relationship, decide on a length of time for your revised agreement. Revisit the agreement periodically.

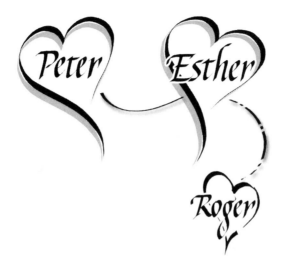

7

Opening Up —
Esther and Peter

*Y*ou're both in your thirties with successful careers. You've been living together for years, without children, and you're happy with your relationship. The only problem is that your partner keeps falling in love with other people. This upsets your relationship every time it happens. You want to trust your partner but it's difficult. Logically, you understand that it's not entirely possible to be attracted to only one person for all of your life. You don't mind your partner's daydreaming, and you've gotten used to her close and sometimes flirtatious contacts with her extended circle of friends. Rationally, you understand that this is who she is, but emotionally it's more of a problem since you suffer from severe bouts of jealousy. You can't bear the thought that at some point your partner might turn her daydreams into reality and actually do something with her feelings for someone else, especially since she's indicated a desire to do just that. These concerns about what the future may hold are creating uncertainty for both of you.

Peter and Esther are grappling with this scenario.

Esther, thirty, and Peter, thirty-four, have been together for twelve years now and are completely comfortable with each other. Life is good. The only recurring issue they have in their relationship is that Esther keeps falling in love with other men. She has

105

a wide social circle and her relationship to some of her friends has, at times, become more intense than purely friendship. For the most part, Esther has kept these feelings to herself, as she has no intention of creating problems in her relationship with Peter. Peter, nonetheless, is aware of what's going on, but doesn't mention it. He simply waits it out and is always happy when these phases end. He is open-minded and tolerant enough, but it is still a relief when things return to normal and Esther no longer daydreams about someone else. For that matter, these periods never last that long, since there is always someone new showing up in Esther's life. If it's not a colleague at work, then it is the guy behind the bar, or at the café, or at the theater who distracts her, or it's the fascinating man she's gotten to know on the Internet. Sometimes it is all too much for Peter. He understands completely that Esther is attracted to other men, and that she has no intention of leaving him. Despite all Esther's feelings for other men, Peter is sure that he is still the most important man in her life. She hasn't had a serious relationship with another man since she and Peter married, but still Peter finds Esther's wandering attractions difficult because, to be blunt, he gets incredibly jealous.

Six months ago, Esther and Peter had weathered a crisis in their relationship when Esther had kissed Roger, a friend from the boat club. Esther told Peter two weeks later when he noticed that she was always chatting online with Roger, and that it was nigh on impossible to distract her attention away from the computer. Peter had been furious when Esther told him about the kiss, and he had to exercise great self-control to keep himself from going out, finding Roger and punching him. That bastard better keep his filthy hands (lips) off Esther! Subsequently, Peter worked off his anger on the tennis court, and later he and Esther talked about it. Peter was upset that Esther waited so long to tell him that she had kissed Roger, and didn't confess right away. It hadn't helped at all when Esther told Peter that she didn't really enjoy the kiss as Roger has a prickly mustache.

A few days later they laughed about it. In his head he could explain to himself that, OK, Esther's in love with someone else, but that doesn't mean that she wants to leave me. Peter understands that such a thing is possible, but emotionally it makes no sense to him. In fact, he had met one of Roger's female friends at a party and chatted with her over cocktails. But Peter was not interested in pursuing the contact as there is only one woman for him, and that woman is Esther. Peter simply is not able to open his heart to anyone else. Esther is different. She sees many different men that seem to have some trait enticing her to fall in love. To make things worse, his trust in Esther took a real knock when he found out that she hid something from him. To help sort this out, Esther and Peter visited Leonie.

A firm foundation

When Esther and Peter stepped into my practice I saw a solid couple that got on well with each other. At first glance there didn't seem to be any tension between them at all. Peter spoke first. Occasionally, as Peter was speaking, Esther interrupted to try to explain something or to fill in a detail, but each time Peter quickly resumed speaking.

In fact, I noticed that they never seemed to let each other finish speaking. When Peter was done with the story, I asked them both what they wanted to achieve with the coaching from me. Peter said that he felt very unsure when he thought of the future. Esther had never had an affair, but he was relatively sure it could happen. He wanted to learn how to deal with his uncertainty and he wanted to get his jealousy under control. Esther supported this completely. It would be really great if Peter wasn't so jealous. Although they seemed to be able to talk about what was happening it never seemed to cure his jealousy. In their quest to come to grips with the situation, they'd read a number of articles about polyamory. What they read really spoke to them and they had recognized themselves in the material. Esther had discovered that she really isn't monogamous, even though she is in a monogamous relationship, and she even thought that she might be polyamorous. She would really like (albeit in the future) to be able to do something with her feelings for other men. At the moment she is allowing herself to be held back by Peter's jealousy and her own uncertainty. Although there is no panic about it, she could also imagine that at some point she would want to express her feelings for other men physically as well. However if Peter is so incredibly jealous then she will simply continue to push that to some unknown future point, as she doesn't want to lose him. She can't imagine life without him. On his side, Peter said that he didn't want to be jealous and would really like to simply be able to be happy for her. They had indeed often talked of this as the ideal outcome.

Peter had also read about "compersion," a newly coined term that describes a feeling of empathetic happiness that we can feel when our partners experience happiness and joy with someone else. He thought that was a great theory, but couldn't imagine ever experiencing it in reality. At the moment, the only thing he feels is jealousy, nothing else. Esther and Peter wondered if it would be possible to open their relationship in the future, or whether such an attempt would be doomed to failure. I complimented them for the courage they displayed in being willing to talk about such an option for their relationship. By being willing to explore options they could then make the best choice for them.

To find an answer to their question we needed to first understand the fundamentals of their relationship. How are they investing in their relationship and how could they strengthen the trust between them?

Opening up a relationship

Most of us have only one "closed" i.e. monogamous, intimate relationship at any given time. On the other hand some of us have "open" i.e. non-monogamous relationships. In these open relationships each partner has the freedom to share intimacy with other people, with the full awareness and permission of their partners. The basis of an open relationship, therefore, is honesty and transparency with all concerned parties. What exactly the intimacy with other people entails depends on our wishes and desires. Some of us are just looking to flirt, while others of us may want to have close, intimate friendships with other men or women. Some want to be able to go out on dates where we can flirt, kiss or maybe do more. Yet others are looking for couples to have an erotic evening with at home or to go to a swingers club together. What for some of us is a bridge too far is simply the first step for others. Some of us open up our relationships to allow ongoing complementary relationships with other people. Those of us who identify as polyamorous often would like to be able to express our love for others in many different ways. In short: an open relationship is a relationship where there are more possibilities than simply "you and me." What "open" means is something we decide for ourselves.

Opening up a relationship is not something that is normally done on a whim. It's not a decision we make one Saturday evening and by the next Friday we're ready to go. Many couples talk about it but don't dare put it into practice out of fear for the impact on their relationship. Other couples discuss it with each other for years before they decide to stretch their relationship boundaries. Even then it can often take months or years before the partners involved find the optimal way to maintain their open relationship. It is a process that can bring renewed passion, fun and exciting times into a relationship. It can also bring challenges that really test a relationship. In other words, opening up a relationship can take time and energy and it requires care to make sure that disappointments are avoided or dealt with.

Before embarking on the journey towards an open relationship, it's important that we feel good about ourselves, that our existing relationships work well, and that we and our partners can fall back on each other and support each other when required. It's essential that we keep talking to our partners if problems or challenges appear. When we open up our relationships, we set not only ourselves in motion, but also our relationships and as a result we can run into some serious challenges. The pitfalls and the not-so-fun parts of ourselves, our partners and our combined behaviors are often exaggerated when complementary relationships exist. This can dramatically affect how we view ourselves, our partners and our relationships. If our relationships are built on solid foundations it can make all the difference when we need to deal with this and other possible challenges.

Successful strategies for sustainable relationships

The following strategies are important in any relationship, whether monogamous or not, but are indispensable for maintaining an open relationship.

- Ensure that you communicate well. Use "I" statements and don't blame others. Listen actively (see chapter three for more about active listening).
- Develop a good relationship with yourself. Work on knowing who you really are. What are your qualities? What are your blind spots? Ensure that you enjoy being with yourself and that you can happily be alone.
- Ensure that you and your partner feel safe with each other. Trust yourself, accept yourself and dare to be yourself. Accept each other as you

are and be aware of each other's differences. When there is trust and safety you can allow yourself to be vulnerable with each other, which increases the intimacy between you.

+ Give each other your complete attention. Be completely there for each other when you spend time together and avoid distractions.
+ Invest in each other and plan to spend time together on a regular basis. You are not just parents, colleagues or friends. You are, above all, partners.
+ Stay in touch with your sexuality and be upfront about your wishes and needs.
+ Keep it exciting, surprise each other regularly. That way you keep the relationship alive.
+ Treat your partner as your best friend. Respect each other and each other's unique qualities.
+ Stay interesting. Maintain your identity and be autonomous.
+ Know what you want and what you don't want and make this clear. Make conscious choices and listen to your own internal sense of what's right or not.
+ Evaluate your relationship regularly. Pay special attention to each other's needs and desires when you do this. Are you still practicing what is important for you both as individuals and as a relationship?

During their first session, Peter and Esther examined their connections to each other using a connection wheel (see chapter 1) and the "Connection Cards" from *The Relationship Game*. I then let them explain to each other what the connections they had chosen meant. They were both surprised when it turned out that each of them had very different meanings associated with the Feel Safe With Each Other card, which they both chose. For Peter, the word "safety" was connected to care and protection. He felt good being with Esther and thought it was wonderful that they cared for each other when necessary and that he could protect her. Esther, on the other hand, associated safety with being able to truly be herself without being judged. She admitted that she did not always feel safe with Peter. Peter was shocked when he heard this, as he had never expected that she would feel inhibited about telling him about her feelings. This gave him food for thought.

As the session progressed, I noticed that Esther and Peter had a tendency to bring out each other's negative aspects. She was sometimes quite spiteful and he was at times rather whiney and controlling. I mentioned this gently to them, but then immediately asked them what they liked about each other. Why did they fall for each other in the first place? What made their partner attractive? They looked at each other and started to laugh. Esther said, "We simply have fun with each other. I can laugh with him and I feel so comfortable when he's around." Peter named something similar: "Esther can be so spontaneous and a bit naive sometimes, I love that. I feel at home with her." I then gave them some tasks to do at home. I asked them to note down every day what they appreciated in each other, what things about the other person made them happy and what they enjoyed in each other. They should each make their own list and bring it with them to the next session.

Habits and taking each other for granted

When we've been in a relationship for a while we can begin to take it for granted. Our partners are simply parts of our lives just like jobs, furnishings, meals and televisions. Many partners become so used to each other that they are no longer aware of what they value in each other. The initial spark between them has long gone and what was once attractive can slowly turn into irritations. This is what had happened to Esther and Peter.

The next time I saw Esther and Peter they were elated. They'd both worked really hard on their tasks and were very curious to find out about each other's lists. Esther had written that she found it wonderful that Peter was so caring. When she came home exhausted from work one evening he ran her a warm bath and brought her a glass of wine. She was used to him doing this but realized when she thought about it that it was a really special thing for him to do. She also noted that when she'd had a problem at work last week, he'd been very supportive. He helped her think through the best way to deal with the problem and had searched for some relevant information on the Internet for her. She had really appreciated that as Peter is especially good with the computer. She also likes the fact that he is so cuddly and that he played with her hair as she sat next to him on the couch. She likes the fact that she can talk to him about almost any subject. When they read the paper together on Saturday mornings she enjoys discussing the news with him. He is always interested in what is happening in the world. Peter had also fixed the lamp in the bathroom right away when it broke, he's very handy. She only needed to ask for help once and it was done. She really appreciated that about him.

Peter also made a list. He enjoyed it when Esther ran through the house singing, she is always so cheery. He thought it was wonderful that Esther always has such great ideas for their holidays. She is always up for fun trips to faraway places. He is impressed by her large circle of friends; it is obvious that Esther has a big heart and cares for the people around her. She is totally present and really wants to be there for all the people that are important to her. Peter also appreciates the fact that she never causes a fuss if he wants to go spend a weekend with his friends. He finds it very touching that she gets so emotional when they watch a film or drama series on TV, as he's a bit more restrained. He really loves her cooking and she always comes up with new recipes. It was wonderful to see how delighted and excited Peter and Esther's reactions were when they heard each other's lists. "You know what, we do all these things for each other but seldom appreciate each other. We just take each other for granted!"

In the rest of the session, we looked at how they behave with each other using the "Behavior Cards" from *The Relationship Game*. I asked them each to choose ten cards that represent the most important behaviors they think should be present in their ideal relationship. Afterwards we looked at whether they were aware of each other's wishes in this area and how their wishes differ. We also made a survey of which aspects are present in their relationship, which ones aren't and which ones can be improved. Sometimes, when we reached certain cards we stopped and worked with them for quite a while in order to consider the behavior that was highlighted. For instance, they both found the card Give Each Other Space And Freedom important. Peter thought that Esther was very good at that, while Esther felt that the way Peter gave her space could be improved. He had a strong tendency to want to be in control and she felt that he often pried for too many details about her feelings of love for others. Peter found the Be Open And Honest With Each Other card very important and had the feeling that Esther was not open enough with him when she was in love with someone else. Esther volunteered that she felt Peter didn't really listen to her but instead always countered with comments insofar as she simply kept things to herself instead of having to deal with Peter's retorts. We agreed to look at this communication dynamic in a following session.

They then looked at having fun together, which was important for both of them. Right now, their individual interests — like sports or computer activities — keep them apart. They both chose the Give Compliments Or Show Appreciation card, and their exercise at home had made it clear to them that complementing was something they'd like to continue.

Invest in your relationship

Not all of us are used to investing in our relationships. In fact, many people consider their relationship's highpoint to be their wedding day. Months of preparation, and a great deal of money go into making an unforgettable day, with the honeymoon as the final touch. It almost seems like the wedding day itself is the final goal. Afterwards, the rest of the world demands attention: work, civic duties, social life and social causes, hobbies and, of course, the children. As we focus on day-to-day concerns, it is easy to neglect our relationships. The problem is that it's *after* the wedding that the real work in a relationship begins. There would probably be a much higher rate of successful marriages if we invested more time and money in marital maintenance, rather that spending it all on the ceremony. Taking stock of our relationship with a view to making improvements is not something we're used to doing, but it is one of the most effective ways to prevent divorce.

Peter and Esther immediately saw the impact of taking a good hard look at their relationship. They became aware again of each other's positive qualities and they started to appreciate each other more. They decided to reevaluate their communication patterns and the ways these behaviors influence their relationship. In the following session we paid attention to the way Esther and Peter communicate. We did this using two communication tools: the "listening survey" and the "speaking survey."

The communication surveys

The ability to listen well is a crucial relationship skill. In my practice, I like to use a tool called the "listening survey" to help people understand how they listen to other people and to pinpoint areas for improvement. Some of the questions in the survey are:

- Are you often busy thinking of an answer while your partner is speaking?
- Do you try to see things from your partner's point of view?
- Do you try to find an answer whenever your partner tells you something?

After a client fills in the survey, I ask him or her to look closely at the responses, and to think about his or her way of listening. I then ask the client to imagine what his or her partner might think about this way of listening, and to note where he or she might want to pay special attention over the next few weeks. His or her partner does the same. They then compare notes with each other to discover if there are any surprises, and to choose some specific points to work on. Ultimately, of course, it is important that each partner takes responsibility for his or her own side of the communications equation.

When Esther looked at her completed listening survey she saw that she often was busy thinking of other things when Peter was talking to her. She also realized that she found it quite difficult to stay focused on him and whatever he was talking about. That was a blind spot for her. On his side, Peter discovered that he had the tendency to constantly interrupt Esther and offer immediate solutions that she was not asking for. Instead, Esther often just wanted to tell her story and talk herself through a problem. She often found her own solutions that way.

Esther and Peter realized that they could improve their communication and both came up with their own suggestions for what they could each do. Esther said that she would do her best to be fully present and pay full attention to Peter when he was talking, and to put her own thoughts to one side as he spoke. If she did find that her thoughts were wandering she would tell him, so, if necessary, he could backtrack and repeat himself to ensure that she heard the whole story. Peter offered to stop offering solutions all the time, and to let Esther know that he was really listening to her by looking at her when she speaks.

When I saw them two weeks later they told me that their communication had improved and that they felt that they understood each other much better now. We then looked at the way they spoke to each other using the "speaking survey." The speaking survey works the same way as the listening survey except that the questions are all about the way we talk to each other. Esther discovered that she tends to talk a great deal but that she finds it difficult to get to the point. Peter offered to help by listening better, summarizing what she is saying regularly and to ask questions without offering his own solutions at the same time. Peter noticed that he is often quite critical towards Esther and promised to not be as quick to voice his opinion or judgement. Peter also observed that he finds it easier to express his feelings by doing rather than speaking. Esther offered to ask Peter about what he feels and to show him more appreciation so that it is easier for him to be open to her.

Improving communication

It takes time to make improvements to the way we communicate. It can't be done all at once. It's virtually impossible to work effectively on all the facets of our communication simultaneously and anyway many of the patterns we are stuck in creep back into our interactions quite quickly. It is quite difficult to break the circles we get stuck in, and to replace them with positive behavior. One way to help do this is to focus on one particular aspect of our way of communicating and do our best to change just that. If we want to learn a new way of doing something, we have to repeat it many times in order for it to stick and become habitual. For example, if we're not used to giving compliments, then it is a real art to learn to be aware of the exact moment when a compliment should be delivered (as it can be counter productive to do so at the wrong moment). When we master one aspect, we can then move onto the next skill that needs attention.

Esther and Peter worked for the next few months on the way they communicate and the way they express appreciation for each other. They noticed that their bond to each other strengthened during this time and that the level of trust in the relationship grew. Only then did they feel they were ready to go back and look at their original request for assistance: How can we deal with the fact that Esther keeps falling in love and that Peter is so jealous?

It turned out that the thing Peter had the most difficulty with when it came to his jealousy was his inability to separate his thoughts from his feelings. Rationally he was prepared to allow Esther to be in love with other people, and would be very happy if he could be a bit more relaxed and free about it. In practice, though, nothing ever came of this as his feelings of jealousy were far too overwhelming and painful. When he discovered that Esther had kissed someone else, he couldn't contain himself. His anger and aggression surprised not only Esther, but also himself. He hated himself for it and wished from the bottom of his heart that he could change.

POLYAMORY DEFINED

Polyamory (often abbreviated to 'poly') is a word coined in the United States in the early 1990s. It is a hybrid word (from the Greek πολυ [poly,] meaning many or several, and the Latin *amor* [love]). It is most often used to refer to the practice of having more than one intimate relationship at a time with the full knowledge and consent of everyone involved. The relationships can be sexual or non-sexual but by definition they are always based on a loving connection between the partners. Sex-only relationships are, by definition, not expressions of polyamory.

Polyamory is quite different from the other forms of multi-partner relationships that have existed for thousands of years. The most common historical forms of polygamy (relationships with more than two partners) are polygyny (one man, many wives) and, less commonly, polyandry (one wife, many husbands). Both of these variants were usually practiced in a strictly hierarchical manner, however. In contrast, the idea of polyamory places great emphasis on equality and most people would, for instance, not consider a traditional Mormon polygamous household polyamorous.

People who self-identify as polyamorous tend to value honesty, integrity and transparency very highly. They also often view polyamory not so much as a behavioral choice but instead as part of who they are. Being polyamorous is a completely separate issue from choosing to live a polyamorous lifestyle. For instance, someone who considers themselves polyamorous and yet chooses to live in a monogamous relationship is still polyamorous, they're simply choosing not to express that facet of their being. Increasingly, polyamorous people are choosing to openly explore the world of multiple relationships. For some, this means negotiating a new agreement within an existing monogamous relationship to allow each partner to maintain other intimate relationships while continuing to keep their "primary" relationships at the center of their lives. Other people choose to have multiple partners and may live alone, with some, or indeed with all of their partners. There are many variations of polyamorous practices, and many people find that their personal expressions of polyamory change over time. A not uncommon scenario is that a couple might choose to explore relationships with a number of other people over a period of time and then settle down with one or two of these "secondary" partners. There is no fixed model for polyamory.

One of the most difficult concepts that many polyamorous people often struggle to convey to others is the idea that simply because someone is polyamorous it does not mean that they "sleep around" or are open to short-term sexual encounters. Just the opposite is often the case — polyamory is about love after all, and loving relationships often take time to develop and blossom. In other words, if someone says they are polyamorous it would be unwise to make any assumptions as to how they live their lives and, crucially, it says nothing about how they might wish to interact with other people (or us!). As so many poly people say, "Just because I'm poly it doesn't mean I want to have sex with you."

We don't know how many people consider themselves polyamorous but estimates range from two to thirty percent of the adult population. To illustrate the difficulty in obtaining an accurate figure, one can consider a common discussion that is often held about polyamory versus cheating. Some people claim that the reason cheating is so widespread is that many people are polyamorous but don't realize or acknowledge it. On the other hand, others say that people who cheat are behaving in ways that are in total opposition to everything polyamorous people value highly (like honesty). Without doubt, the number of articles, TV programs, workshops, conferences and events about polyamory are increasing exponentially. The concept of polyamory is clearly something that is helping more and more people make sense of their feelings of love for more than one person.

Dealing with jealousy

Life is not richer by being free of emotions,
but rather by being free to deal with them.
—ANDRÉ LASCARIS

Jealousy is almost always present in relationships, especially when other people come into the picture, such as in an open relationship. It is a very human emotion that a great many people suffer from and find very difficult to deal with. The reason for this is that jealousy is not just one emotion but is instead a collection of feelings that arise out of negative thoughts and associated fears. This complexity reflects itself in the different ways there are to deal with it. Here are some of the most common strategies:

EMBRACE OUR JEALOUSY

Feelings of jealousy can be strong, violent and quite unpleasant. As a result we often try to resist them. This usually does not help. Our feelings are only reinforced this way. One of the first steps in learning to deal with jealousy is to accept that these feelings simply are there, to allow ourselves to experience our feelings of fear and pain and not to run away from them. Negative emotions are a part of life and being human. Our feelings of jealousy are normal, they're allowed to be, and we can simply accept them. Breathe into them when we feel them in our bodies. View ourselves with love and respect even when jealousy threatens to take hold. Remember that we *have* feelings, but we are not our feelings.

BE AWARE OF AND MANAGE OUR THOUGHTS

Jealousy is a complex collection of fears, negative emotions and negative thoughts. As a result, dealing with jealousy can be a time-consuming process. One of the ways to do this intellectually is to analyze what is happening and look at the different components one by one. If we can be aware of what triggers our jealousy, *when it happens*, we can become conscious of the thoughts, feelings and emotions that arise *in that instant* and work with those emotions consciously. As an example, I might imagine that my partner is sharing an intimate kiss with someone else. How might I respond if I see it or hear about it later? I might want, just like Peter, to physically attack the other person. It's logical: something happens, we feel jealous and from a feeling of anger we act. Yet between the event and the reaction a great deal takes place inside of us. All sorts of thoughts, many unconscious, stream through us and trigger associated feelings and emotions. For instance, when I see my partner kiss someone else, I might think "I'm not allowed to exist" or "I'm not attractive" or "I'm not good enough." This type of reaction can cause us to feel unsure or unimportant which then translates into jealousy.

Therefore, one way to get a grip on jealousy is to question our thoughts: "Is it really true that I am not attractive? How can I be sure that I am not attractive?" followed by "How would I react if I didn't have that thought?" Once we've become aware of our thought processes we can then formulate positive and supportive thoughts (affirmations) to counteract these negative thoughts. In this case we might use "I'm special in my own way and attractive to my partner," or "I am unique and I have a lot to offer to my partner." Sometimes it helps to say these affirmations aloud or to repeat them to ourselves.

This process takes courage and awareness. So many of the thoughts that we have about relationships stem from common monogamous assumptions such as "he's mine" or "my partner is here to make me happy." When an event occurs that threatens one of these assumptions the reaction can be swift and powerful. It's not always easy to isolate the individual components triggered when this happens, or to be fully aware of what these particular emotions, feelings or thoughts are. Indeed, when we embark on this process we often realize that our entire relationship paradigms are based on romantic ideals of "two against the world," which are unrealistic and flawed. If we want to consciously explore opening relationships we need to be prepared to confront this paradigm shift head on, and step by step.

UNDERSTAND OUR FEARS

Fears have a purpose: they alert us to potential danger. Fear is a natural survival mechanism, and we all have it to varying degrees. However, it seems that often we feel as much as twice the fear that is warranted for a certain threatening situation. So next time we feel fear we could consider this: "I feel very fearful, but half this fear will be enough." How would we react if we were only half as fearful?

There are many kinds of fears hidden underneath jealousy such as the fear of:

- not being good enough
- losing our partner
- abandonment
- that someone else is better in bed than we are

All of these fears can be deeply upsetting and that is completely normal. However, if we react based on fears of what might happen, then we're creating negative pictures of the future. The more we feed our pictures with our thoughts, the stronger the associated emotions become. If we're not careful we can end up with self-fulling prophecies as our negativities can precipitate the very events that we fear so much.

As an antidote to this scenario we can try to imagine not being affected by jealousy at all. We might imagine reacting from positive points of view — positive pictures of the future. What would a worldview based on a lack of fear look like?

We can choose how to react and whether or not to let our fears get the better of us. Of course, detrimental events happen and our fears can be useful warnings. However, jealous fears cannot only be exaggerated way out of proportion, they can create the very situation we are most afraid of. Choosing to act consciously from a known place, rather than a place of unnamed fear is one of the most potent tools in conquering jealousy.

DISCOVER OUR UNDERLYING NEEDS

The great thing about negative feelings and fears is that there are always desires or needs hidden under them, waiting to be discovered. For instance, under the fear of being abandoned may well be a need for affirmation and appreciation. Beneath anger there may be a hidden need to stand up for personal boundaries. A fear of losing someone may conceal a need for reassurance. A need to control may indicate a need to release or to surrender. Under the fear of not being good enough may lie the need to mean something to someone else or a desire for more self-confidence and this, in its turn, is something we can then develop. If we know what our underlying needs are, we can also come up with ways of meeting them. Sometimes others can help — such as needs for acknowledgement. Other times, we can meet our own needs — such as improving self-confidence. When we meet our needs, our feelings of jealousy slowly subside.

CHOOSE TO BEHAVE DIFFERENTLY

Many of our reactions are habitual and we are not always aware of what we do. Becoming aware of why we do what we do and learning how to change the thoughts that drive our actions is one way of getting our negative reactions under control. We can also simply do something else when we feel jealousy beginning to take control. For instance, consider the example of someone experimenting with an open relationship, and their partner is out on date with someone else. If a feeling of jealousy comes on, then instead of creeping into bed and hiding under the covers he or she can choose to see a play. Following this example, we can go see friends, watch films, stay home and work on a project… generally do something we enjoy when our partners are out. If we find ourselves getting angry and picking fights with our partners, we can learn to count to ten, and then manage our anger differently — like go running or exercising. With practice, we can work on being autonomous and being fair to ourselves instead of acting out.

UNDERSTANDING AND WORKING THROUGH OLD PAIN

Jealousy is not only triggered by underlying emotions such as fear but also by things that have happened to us in the past, events which often have no direct connection to our present situation. In this way, jealousy can serve us well by making us aware of traumatic events from our pasts that are still significantly affecting our lives. Sometimes, simply being aware of this coupling can be enough to release the grip of old trauma. Sometimes, we need to go back and identify what happened, and take steps to undo the damage that was caused to our emotional and energetic systems.

One way to work through old pain is to use techniques such as guided visualization. This technique is often used by coaches to analyze and change feelings of jealousy and the behavior associated with it. This involves imagining, in great detail, a situation where feelings of jealousy are strongest and then examining those feelings, fears and negative thoughts with a conscious intent to replace them with positive thoughts. Learning how to deal with jealousy can be an incredible gift that allows us to develop a whole new view of ourselves and our relationship(s).

Peter found it difficult to figure out how to deal with his jealousy. I suggested to him that we work on this in a separate guided visualization session with him alone. This way he would have time and space to look at his feelings, thoughts and fears. We agreed that he would tell Esther about the exercise and the results. At the start of the guided visualization session, Peter spoke of his hesitation and concerns about the exercise. He was afraid that his emotions would be too strong for him. I explained to Peter that he could stop the "film" at any time during the visualization. He could also turn off the sound or he could watch in black and white. If he chose to stop the visualization, he didn't have to immediately start it again. He could take a break. That reassured him. He decided to have me narrate the visualization without sound, in other words I would only describe scenes to him without any dialogue from the "actors." After each scene I would then ask him some questions.

We then started the visualization with a scene that featured Esther meeting a man she has fallen in love with. Peter burst into tears when we reached the part where Esther kisses her so-called "lover" and gazes passionately into his eyes as he asks her to leave Peter. We stopped the film at that point and looked at Peter's thoughts and feelings during the visualization. He was full of anger, sadness, fear and despair. He thought: "I'm not good enough," "she's abandoning me" and "he is better than I am." I wrote these thoughts down so we could come back to them later and reword them into positive, supportive affirmations. We then took a closer look at Peter's fears.

When he looked deeper, Peter saw that his deepest fear was abandonment, followed by his concern that he would no longer be the only man in Esther's life. He was also very afraid of losing control.

I asked Peter if his fear of abandonment could be connected to something in his past. What was his childhood like? What was it like growing up? How close was he to his parents? Peter explained that his father had left their family when Peter was ten. His father had a girlfriend at the time and his parents divorced soon afterwards. Although his father had promised him that they would stay in contact, Peter saw very little of him after the divorce. His father started a new family and put all of his attention there instead. When Peter visited his father, Peter often felt like there was no room for him. This was especially hard for him when he saw what a great time his new halfbrother had with his father and his father's wife. When Peter told me about this he became quite emotional. He'd suppressed his awareness of his feelings long ago and he had not spoken of it for ages. I suggested that we have a look at dealing with his past and that he could try to find out when he first felt the feelings "I'm being abandoned" and "I'm not good enough." He started on this task by using the "letter to yourself" exercise. In this exercise, I asked him to write a compassionate letter to his younger self — to the ten year old boy who had experienced such a hard time when his father left. In the letter, I also asked him to tell his younger self what he would have wished for him.

In the following session, I worked further with Peter on releasing his old pain. Writing the letter had brought many emotions and feelings to the surface, and he felt good about giving himself the love, support and acknowledgement that he had not received as a child.

We continued to look at Peter as he is now and to see how he could use his inherent positive qualities to work constructively with his current situation. To do this, I let Peter make physical contact with all the different parts of himself by asking him to create a sub-personality for each of his qualities. For instance, Peter can be very relaxed and easygoing, so that sub-personality might be imagined as Peter sitting in a comfortable chair in a café, sipping his favorite drink and simply enjoying watching the world go by.

To find out what wisdom the easy-going Peter has to offer himself, I suggested that Peter sit on a different chair. I then asked him pretend he was looking back at himself, and speaking from the point of view of the easygoing sub-personality to give himself some advice. He gave himself the advice to simply trust himself and relax a bit more. We then repeated this exercise with some of the other traits, and Peter soon realized that he already owns the bulk of the skills and knowledge he needs. The reason he couldn't access this wisdom was simply that the pain from his past was reasserting itself as jealousy in the present, and it was getting in the way. Although it had been difficult and unpleasant for Peter to go back and look at this past, it had ultimately helped him to discover that underneath his jealousy was the pain from his childhood, and by releasing it, he'd find the skills he needed for the present.

Not everyone who suffers from jealousy is prepared to work through the pain of their past. Sometimes there are other things that we need to do before we can tackle such issues. Everyone has their own pace and chooses their own timing. There are many methods that therapists and coaches use to teach us how to deal with the pain from our past. The letter-writing exercise is one. Another one is the life-schema exercise discussed in chapter one.

Something we all face when trying to move forward, past pain or not, is the presence of our Inner Critic, or our processes of internal negative self-reinforcement, which can make it very difficult to move forward into new behaviors and thought patterns. A crucial skill to develop, therefore, is the art of quieting our Inner Critic. There are countless books, articles and techniques available on how to do this and finding one that works can be useful.

Peter had talked extensively with Esther about our sessions and the way his past was affecting his current feelings. As he did this he began to notice that his feelings of jealousy were still there but that he could manage them much better. He could talk to Esther about what had happened without getting instantly angry or aggressive. This was a major step forward for both of them. As their communication improved so too did their ability to talk about Esther's polyamory. She knows now that she can be more herself, and that Peter is truly open to giving her more space. Their mutual trust in the future of their relationship grew dramatically.

After Peter's hard work on his jealousy I took another look with both of them at their current situation and the way they might deal with Esther's polyamorous feelings. She still has feelings for Roger and wants to develop this new relationship if possible. Esther suggested that she and Peter would make a date with Roger and his woman friend so that they could all discuss this in the open. Peter was amenable to the idea. He really liked the idea of being present when Esther and Roger talk about what they might do together. This gave him a feeling of safety and he liked the idea that he might be able to give some input and even voice any concerns he might have. And, to be totally honest, he was also a bit curious to see that interesting friend of Roger's again and to see how he felt about her. Both Peter and Esther had the feeling that they were ready for a new dimension in their relationship and looked forward to getting started.

> *Make sure to create space to breathe.*
> *The more we try to overcome our fear through clinging on to others,*
> *the more our fear is confirmed, and the other will indeed leave us.*
> —ANSELM GRÜN

Questions you can ask yourself

+ How do I deal with my feelings for someone other than my partner?
+ How do I talk about others with my partner and what are our agreements?
+ How do I deal with feelings of jealousy?
+ What is my greatest fear for my relationship? What is my underlying need? How can I meet this need?
+ What part of my jealousy is related to pain from my past? What messages did I receive from my parents or caretakers that my jealousy is stimulating?
+ What do I need to be able to stretch my limits? What steps would I like to take?

Tips for expanding the limits of your relationship

+ Accept that stretching the limits of your relationship can be scary but also exciting. Fear is simply a normal part of the equation.
+ Don't let yourself be paralyzed by fear. Growth is all about feeling fear and taking a step forward anyway. There is no such thing as a mistake, simply a new experience to learn from.
+ Make clear agreements about your boundaries. What do you want and what don't you want? Respect each other's boundaries.
+ Live as much as possible in the here and now and stop worrying about what might happen in the future. Be fully present with yourself and the moment and say "yes" to the present. Focus your attention on the things that you can influence yourself.
+ Invest in your development and growth. Take responsibility for your own happiness.
+ Take into account your partner's pace. Let the person who moves slowest be the one that sets the pace, but make sure, on the other hand, that you keep moving.
+ Maintain your sense of humor. The ability to see the funny side of yourself and your situation can be freeing and provides perspective.
+ Make sure to have fun and do interesting things not only with your new love, but also with your partner. Keep investing in your main relationship. Let your partner know how special he or she is to you and why.
+ A relationship that is opening up is a relationship in movement. Wishes and needs can change over time. Take time to evaluate these with each other on a regular basis.

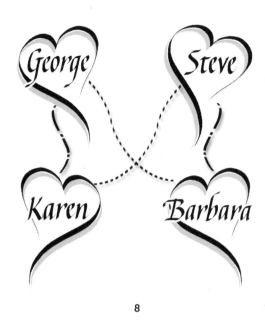

8

Swinging:
Stretching Sexual Boundaries —
Karen and George

*Y*ou've been together for quite a few years now, you have a child and your life is settled. *You lead a monogamous lifestyle and have a satisfactory sex life. Satisfactory, but to be blunt, that's about it. At this point, you know each other very well, and your passion has pretty much disappeared over the years. Secretly, you long for something new. You've heard about swinging — an activity that can spice up your sex life by having sexual or erotic contact with other like-minded couples. You think that this might be something for you, but at the same time you are scared. How do you start and what can you expect? How can you make sure that your primary relationship isn't negatively affected? How do you avoid problems?*

Karen and George are curious too.

Karen, thirty-six, and George, thirty-nine, have known each other for thirteen years. They are a married couple with one child. They have both been with other lovers, but have lived monogamously since their marriage. One evening, they watched a TV program about swinging which sparked a long discussion between them. Would this be something for them? George liked the idea, but Karen wasn't so sure. In any case, they decided that a bit more information couldn't hurt, so they decided to research the possibilities — first by searching on the Internet. They discovered that there are lots of swingers clubs, and many organize special couples-only evenings. The idea, they read, involves meeting other couples and, if it clicked between you and one of them, you enjoy an erotic evening together. Although it sounded exciting, they found that it was difficult to take the next step and visit a club. What would be the consequences if they decided to open up their relationship sexually? How could they keep it all under control so that their relationship would not be threatened? They were unsure, and decided that a visit to a relationship coach might be a good next step.

Unexpected results

When I met George and Karen, I quickly realized that they are a couple who are used to communicating and who can talk openly with each other about their sexuality. In our introductory session, Karen and George spoke extensively about their relationship, how they had met each other, and why they had decided to contact me. They had many friends but found it difficult to talk with any of them about the fact that they were curious to learn more about swinging. They were clearly relieved to have found an impartial place to share their ideas and questions.

It was clear to me that George and Karen have a stabile relationship and playing the *Relationship Game* with them revealed that it was indeed based on a solid foundation. Karen and George enjoyed having this confirmed. With the help of the "Behavior Cards" we examined the ten aspects they both felt that they would want to consider if they were to invite other people to interact with them sexually. They chose the following cards together:

1. Maintain A Sexual Relationship
2. Be Open And Honest with Each Other
3. Have Fun Together
4. Communicate Wishes And Needs
5. Listen To Each Other
6. Take Each Other's Feelings And Opinions Seriously
7. Indicate Boundaries And Limits
8. Encourage Or Challenge Each Other
9. Give Each Other Space And Freedom
10. Honor Agreements And Promises

We looked at why George and Karen felt that these cards were important for them to ensure they both shared the same understanding. In addition to the ten cards, they both mentioned that practicing safe sex was very important. I asked George and Karen to each make a list of their own sexual desires and fantasies, and to indicate which ones they would most like to experience. After that, I asked them to exchange lists. Then, they could talk with each other about what they would like to try in reality and what they would absolutely not want to do.

George then asked me more about swingers clubs. They both wanted to know more about what happens there. What could they expect if they went to one? I started to tell them what I knew. Soon, George stopped me, and said that he'd heard enough. He wanted to find out more first hand, and Karen agreed. They both were excited by the idea and were keen to visit a club. After they tried it, however, they realized that they reacted differently than they each expected, and came back to talk about it.

If you worry too much about the road
you can sometimes forget to walk.
—JULIET DAVENPORT

Swinging: it's still a taboo

Swinging is a social activity that involves like-minded people having recreational sex with each other. In most countries — and the Netherlands, the US and the UK are no exceptions — swinging is taboo. In the workplace, at cafés or at parties, people will happily tell each other about a great meal that they enjoyed at a new restaurant, or talk about the latest films in town, but we rarely hear about someone's visit to the swingers club. Although sexual and erotic material is fed to us constantly through the media and advertising, a visit to a swingers club is, for most people, something we just don't want to know about. We have difficulty understanding what it would be like or what happens there. Some of us imagine a sinister place full of people in raunchy dress willing to do everything and anything.

This picture couldn't be further from the truth. The reality is that all sorts of people go to swingers clubs. People from all social backgrounds have sex, and that is exactly what you see in a club — a cross-section of society — which is part of what makes visiting a swingers club so interesting. In theory, anyone can go to swingers clubs: your neighbor, your baker, your boss, your colleague....

Many find that a swingers lifestyle is an excellent way to stimulate their sex lives and to make their erotic fantasies come true. Usually, most swingers find falling in love or becoming too intimate emotionally with others threatening for their own relationships, and complementary relationships with those they meet at clubs are out of the question. The relatively anonymous contact that swingers have in clubs makes it easier for them to stretch their personal boundaries and to enrich their sexual relationships. People try out all sorts of things in clubs. Some enjoy watching their partners having sex with someone else, while others invite one or more people to join them in their lovemaking. Some people go to clubs to find out what it's like to have sex with someone of the same sex, to explore their bisexuality, or follow through on their bisexual fantasies. And, many people see swinging as simply an enjoyable and erotic night out.

One of the ways that we can discover what happens in a swingers club is to simply visit one some evening, and have a look at what happens without getting involved in any of the action ourselves. There are many things that can make the evening fun without having to have sex. Usually clubs have rooms where people can have sex either privately or together, but there are also bars, dance floors and food available. Quite often, there are saunas and/or Jacuzzis as well. One thing that is different from a normal night club, however, is that many swingers clubs have a dress code. This usually works so that by a certain hour (say eleven) everyone is encouraged to change into 'sexy' clothing. This can be lingerie, sexy leather or latex, chains or simply nothing at all. Like saunas, everyone is given a key to their own locker when they arrive so that they can store their personal effects securely and change at their leisure. For many people, the idea that they need to change out of their street clothes can feel strange at first. Remember though that everyone who visits the club is there for the same reason so, at that level, everyone is equal. Many people enjoy dressing up in sexy clothes, and many people who go to clubs do so specifically because they like to be seen — and admired — in their sexy outfits.

Before going to a club, it's a good idea to be fully aware of how we experience sex and to be clear about what we want to do, and don't want to do. Everyone responds differently when they witness other people having sex. One person might get very excited and want to join in right away, while another might take some time to get used to it and will watch curiously while staying good and close to their partner. Yet others feel totally intimidated by the sight of so many people having sex. It's good to consider ahead of time how we might react. A good way to avoid disappointment and misunderstandings is to make very clear agreements before we go out. It's also good to know that in swingers clubs there is a very clear and strictly enforced rule that "No means No." In other words, if other people approach with sexual contact in mind a "No" or a simple hand gesture suffices to set a boundary. It is important, therefore, to know what our boundaries are and to be able to set them.

Karen and George summoned their courage and decided to visit an upscale swingers club. They agreed that on the first evening they would simply go and watch. They had a drink at the bar, danced, chatted with some other people and had a meal. Later on in the evening they went upstairs to watch other couples "in action." They were totally amazed at what they saw and couldn't tear their eyes away. When they finally arrived back home, they were both excited and so full of sexual energy that they enjoyed the best sex they'd had in years. Their sex life really took off after that and the following week was incredible. As the weekend approached, they decided to go a step further and this time they would have sex with each other in a room where others couples were also busy with each other. They had yet another fantastic evening at the club and it was a very sexually stimulating experience for both of them. Back home, their sex life continued to blossom and they felt even closer to each other. They also began to feel quite adventurous as a team.

A month later, they visited the club again. They'd decided to continue experimenting and this time they wanted to find out what it would be like to have sexual contact with another couple. They agreed that if they met another couple that they both found suitable they would use a prearranged sign to discreetly signal each other. They agreed that they would be fine with kissing and oral sex but that neither of them would have actual intercourse. That evening, they met a couple in the Jacuzzi, Barbara and Steve, who they immediately got on well with. Steve suggested that they go upstairs to a private room where they could be together without being disturbed. Karen and George agreed and followed Steve and Barbara upstairs, busily chatting on the way there. When they arrived, Steve almost immediately started paying a great deal of attention to Karen, who clearly liked him and responded enthusiastically. George started to get to know Barbara a bit better, but he was much more reserved. George began to feel a bit uneasy as Steve and Karen's sexual encounter unfolded in front of him, but he didn't say anything or disturb them. George also discovered that he had difficulties getting sexually excited with Barbara. Just as he was busy worrying about his own circumstance, he looked over at Steve and Karen again. George had almost never seen Karen so excited. He thought it was great for her, but it was also tough for him. Barbara noticed this and succeeded in directing George's attention away from Karen. Later, they all went downstairs to the bar where they chatted a bit more and exchanged e-mail addresses.

The following morning Karen was still very excited and wanted to have sex with George, but he wasn't in the mood. He reacted with irritation, and didn't even laugh when she made a joke. Karen realized that they needed to talk. It was only then she understood that they had experienced very different scenarios the previous evening. It worked out in the end, right? And, didn't he have a good time with Barbara? The truth for George, however, was that he was in a bit of shock. He was beginning to doubt whether swapping partners, as they had done the evening before, was really something that he felt OK with. The idea had been very exciting, but when it came down to it, he had expected something different. After this conversation, they didn't speak about the subject for a few weeks.

In the meantime, they got an e-mail from Steve and Barbara wanting to know when they were planning to visit the club again. Karen had chatted on-line with Steve once as well and was keen to make a new date, but George was no longer interested in the idea. Karen was totally confused. He was the one that was so full of enthusiasm and whose idea it had been to go to the swingers club first, and Karen had been the one that had hesitated. Now that she was beginning to really enjoy it, he all of sudden had cold feet. They noticed that their different desires were starting to create tension in their relationship. What should they do?

How to enjoy sex in a swingers club

The main reason most people visit swingers clubs is to be sexually stimulated. It can be useful to know, though, that what sexually stimulates men and what stimulates women can be quite different. Men tend to be stimulated visually and react to what they see. Women, on the other hand, tend to react more to smell and sound. If we're going to enjoy going to clubs (and even if we want to enjoy sex at all!) it is useful to cultivate the ability to respond to these stimuli. There are usually many things that need to be in place in order for us to allow ourselves to be stimulated. Many people are quite sensitive to the atmosphere or surroundings they are in. Soft lighting, luxurious sheets, inspiring music and a sensual decor make big differences. It is also important that we feel comfortable being intimate with our partners, that we feel appreciated and respected and that we both feel safe. It helps if we are relaxed and present when we begin to have sex and are not busy thinking about work or family. If we really want to enjoy sex, we need to get out of our heads and be able to surrender to our feelings and bodily sensations.

It's also important that whatever we do, we do it in a way that we enjoy and find pleasurable and safe. However, not everyone can immediately sense what they like or don't like. This means that we need to learn how to make explicit what we want or are looking for. It's usually much easier to do this with a partner than with a stranger at a club. This new person has no idea if we like to be stroked softly or firmly for instance. Do we get excited by soft nibbles on our skin or do we go completely cold when that happens? Some people like to have someone grab ahold of them quite firmly while others enjoy soft, slow seduction. Do we like the way someone kisses, or not? These are all things that play a part in whether we enjoy sex. One way to ensure that we receive what we enjoy most is to encourage someone who is doing something we like, or to say something like "a bit softer would be wonderful." Expressing desires or wishes in a positive fashion encourages our sexual partners to do what we enjoy. If someone touches us somewhere we don't like, we can simply move the hand to a place we do enjoy. Again, communication is key.

A swingers club does not have the same effect on everyone. Often, there are factors that we are not immediately cognizant of — such as our inherent values and norms or self-critical thoughts — that can affect our sexual experiences. Some people even watch themselves from a distance and start to judge themselves. Many people are surprised when these internal processes kick in as they thought they were going to simply have a good time.

Before Karen and George had even begun to tell their story, it was clear to me that something had changed. Whereas last time it had been George who was enthusiastic and who couldn't wait to get started, this time it was Karen who showed impatience. Karen described how she instantly got on with Barbara and Steve and felt she could trust them. However, she was surprised at how quickly it had gone. Steve seemed to know exactly what Karen liked and before she knew it she had completely let herself go. She had really enjoyed it and had been incredibly turned on the whole week thereafter. She noticed the positive effect it had on her level of sexual desire and she was keen on experimenting more.

George had experienced the evening completely differently. He liked Barbara, and Steve was a great guy, but George had been a bit tense when Steve suggested that they go upstairs. George had started to gently touch Barbara when he saw how Steve almost leapt onto a willing and excited Karen. Although Barbara was a very attractive woman, George simply could not get what was going on between Steve and Karen out of his head. Normally, Karen took a fair few minutes to warm up and get going and what he saw now was a completely different woman. He wasn't sure what to think. What is Steve doing to her? What if Steve wants to have intercourse with Karen, and she is so excited that she simply does it? He tried unsuccessfully to catch Karen's eye. George was so concerned about what was going on between Steve and Karen that he didn't really pay any attention to Barbara, and he felt guilty. He couldn't even be a "real man" for Barbara. Barbara realized that George was nervous and tense and tried to get him to relax. Ultimately this turned out to be fun, but as far as George was concerned, that was the end of the club experiment. It was all too complicated and at the end of the day it wasn't worth it.

Releasing expectations

When we have set our expectations too high we can be our own worst enemies as we create our own disappointments. The problem is that we end up reacting to what we think should happen rather than to what occurs in the present. We're busy trying to make our preconceived notions come true and then we're surprised and upset when it doesn't work. So often, we are only satisfied if our fantasies turn out exactly the way we expected. While it is true that the agreements we've made with our partners ahead of time can provide a certain level of clarity and safety, it is simply not possible to predetermine how such an evening is going to play itself out. The best way to succeed, then, is to release our expectations, and simply stay in the present and respond to what happens.

George had conjured many expectations for the evening, but it turned out differently from what he had imagined, despite all the conversations with Karen beforehand. Karen on the other hand had fewer expectations and simply went along to see what would happen. She had been nervous and was initially somewhat resistant, but afterwards she was glad she'd decided to go with George after all. In our coaching session we decided to look a bit further into George's experience. Through a process of asking questions, summarizing, reflecting and continuing to probe further, we obtained more information about the thoughts and feelings that George had experienced that evening. We then examined his thoughts by writing them down in chronological order like this:

1. I hope it goes well — when Steve suggested they go upstairs.
2. I hope she likes me — when he realized that he might have a sexual encounter with Barbara.
3. Can I really trust her? — when he saw Karen getting excited as Steve started touching her.
4. She's not even thinking about me — when he didn't manage to make visual contact with Karen.
5. He's better than I am — when he saw Karen's massive orgasm.
6. If I could only get an erection — when Barbara started to kiss him.

7. Barbara deserves a good time too, am I up to the task? — when Barbara really started to pay attention to him.

George's emotions and feelings as the evening unfolded were: insecurity, performance anxiety, despair, panic, frustration and loneliness.

Karen was shocked when she saw George's list. She had no idea that their encounter with Steve and Barbara had been so upsetting for George. She'd simply enjoyed herself. In all the excitement she had not paid much attention to what was happening with George. When he tried to explain to her what had occurred, Karen felt guilty; however she was so excited about the possibilities of further adventures at the club she'd pushed her guilt feelings to one side. She thought he just needed to get used to the club scene and if they went more often it would sort itself out.

There would be nothing to frighten you
if you refused to be afraid.
—MAHATMA GANDHI

Finding out where boundaries are by crossing them

There are many ways to discover where our personal boundaries lie. We can talk to our partners about what we think would be fun to explore, tell them what our personal fantasies are, and decide what we're going to do and what we're definitely not going to do. These are certainly important discussions as preparation for a visit to a swingers club, but there are always gray zones as things can happen that we have not foreseen and we simply can't always know how we will respond. Fantasy and reality don't always match up when it comes down to it. For instance, we might be very excited to fantasize about someone having forceful sex with us, but in practice we might find it awful. When we are sexually excited, we can find ourselves on erotic voyages of discovery trying all sorts of things, and afterwards wondering if we really wanted to do that at all, and was it really that great anyway?

In fact, some people experience a sort of inner emptiness after they have had sexual contact with someone other than their partners. They miss the intimacy and the love that they express together. They discover that lust is not the only thing required for them to truly enjoy sex. Others find that it's fun to try something out once, but have no need to repeat the experience. And there are, indeed, people who think it's wonderful to be able to express themselves sexually with no inhibitions and see clubs as an integral part of their sex lives. Everyone is different, so if we're really interested in discovering what is true for us, there is one sure way to find out: try it.

Sometimes, when we are testing our boundaries, we cross them. We can't always see ahead of time what's in front of us. When we find that we've crossed our own lines, it is a good idea to reflect on and evaluate what has happened. If something happens that is not exactly what we want, then we can view it as something to learn from — an opportunity to get to know ourselves better. No child learns to bicycle without falling off from time to time. It's part of the learning curve. If we want to know how it feels to ride a mountain bike, we need to start pedaling.

I asked George and Karen what they would do differently if they could redo their evening at the club. George said that he would have told Steve and Barbara about the agreement between him and Karen: no intercourse but anything else. He would also have liked to have had a little bit of intimate time with Karen upstairs first, just a little chat or a cuddle before she got started with Steve. He'd missed having that. I asked him what he would have needed to do to make that happen. George realized that his expectations had again gotten the better of him as he'd assumed that Karen would simply have known that he needed that moment with her. Eventually, George understood that he was responsible for expressing his own needs clearly.

Karen said that ideally she would have liked to have had more eye contact with George. She admitted that as a result of her excitement she completely forgot to do that. It probably would have helped if they had been positioned closer to each other, possibly even within arms length. (George and Barbara had been a few meters away from Steve and Karen in a rather dark room.) In hindsight, Karen realized that her choice to be so far away was maybe not the best idea. She had wanted to give George the space to be with Barbara as she knew how much he'd been looking forward to the evening and she didn't want to get in his way. They had indeed initially said "giving each other space" was really important for both of them.

We then looked again at the thoughts that George had expressed, starting from when Steve had suggested that they go upstairs. I asked George to identify how his underlying needs might have been met if the evening had gone as he initially hoped it would. We started with the tension and uncertainty he had felt during points one (I hope it goes well) and two (I hope she likes me) and he thought that they still would have been there, but might have been less strong had he and Karen been more clear with Steve and Barbara ahead of time. Points three (Can I really trust her?) and four (She's not even thinking about me) where he was no longer sure that he trusted what Steve and Karen were up to, would not have surfaced at all. This would have had a strong influence on points six and seven, regarding his uncertainty around his ability to be a good sexual partner for Barbara. We looked at the underlying need behind point five (I'm sure he's a better lover than I am). George's underlying need, which is affirmation, was met immediately by Karen the moment I mentioned it. "George, you're a fantastic lover and you know that perfectly well. Don't worry. You're wonderful just as you are."

George and Karen decided at the end of the session that they would make another date with Barbara and Steve at the club. They would first have a chat over a drink and talk about their experiences to make sure that they could all enjoy themselves in the future. George and Karen agreed that, despite the initial hiccup, their swinging experience had indeed brought more passion into their sex life. The sexual energy was flowing between them and they both really enjoyed that.

THE SPIRITUAL GROWTH BENEFITS
OF MULTIPLE SEXUAL PARTNERS

To frequently change partners brings increased benefit...
If one constantly has intercourse with the same partner
their ching-ch'i (sexual vitality) will become weak,
and this is not only of no great benefit to you,
but will cause your partner to become thin and emaciated.

—*TAOIST PRIEST CH'ING NU*
(from Secrets of the Jade Chamber, written in c. 980 AD)

Having sex with more than one person, whether consecutively or simultaneously, is nothing new and, in fact, we humans have been doing it from the
beginning of time (if our historical records are to be believed). Our ancestors all had multiple sexual partners in one form or another. Sometimes this
was practiced in ritual ceremonies for religious or spiritual benefit, other
times it was something that benefited the survival of a culture by ensuring
that babies were born, even when a marriage was not fruitful. Some cultures,
notably in the South Pacific, simply accepted that sex was a fun, normal and
healthy part of human existence and maintained a quite relaxed view on who
slept with whom. In one particular island culture, the women were known
to have a very high libido and as a consequence the men of the community
would often go on long fishing trips together simply to get some rest!

This is all in stark contrast to the shame, guilt and general repression
of sex by many organized religions and other "guardians of morality," who
have made it such a challenge to talk, much less act, in an aware, conscious
and congruent fashion about sex. How many couples never talk to each
other about their needs, desires, and/or fantasies? It sometimes seems
that one of the hardest things to do is to engage in conversations with our
partners about something that is fundamental to who we are.

Realistically, sex can get old. If we do the same thing over and over
without variety, whether it be the way we have sex or the kind of food we
eat, we *will* get bored. We enjoy diversity and sex is no exception. No one
gets upset if we change our wardrobes or try new kinds of food once in a
while. But, try telling our friends, families and colleagues that we're wanting a bit of sexual variety after being married for a few years. The reaction
may not be as affirming. However, suppressing the need for variety is not,
ultimately, a healthy solution as the Taoists observed.

So, is the solution simply to drop all of our inhibitions and moral ideals
and have a sexual free-for-all? That would appear, historically, not to have

been the case in most sex-positive cultures and traditions. These ancient traditions, while on the one hand recognized the need for variety, also had many ways to prepare individuals in order for them to fully enjoy the fruits of their sexuality.

In some cultures, sexual skill and awareness is included in the rites-of-passage for both male and females. There is a West African community, for instance, where young men are instructed by mature women in the art of love, and a young man may not marry until he can demonstrate his ability to bring a woman to orgasm.

Developed, conscious sexuality practices, such as the Taoist and Tantric ones had temples where sex between multiple, or at least alternate, partners was practiced. However, if one delves a bit deeper it becomes apparent that it was not simply a case of "I'm interested in some sex tonight, let's pop down to the temple." On the contrary, at least two years of solid preparation, most of it solo, was required before one could participate in the rites which took place under the guidance of trained (mostly female) masters. This preparation was all about learning to take responsibility for ones own sexuality and to learn to be aware of — and then to be able to guide — the flow of sexual energy in ones own body. Both Taoist and the Tantric texts indicate that orgasmic energy can be circulated and stored. The purpose of these rites was to give the participants an opportunity to refine, or raise the vibrational level of their self-directed sexual energies together with similarly trained adepts.

So, paradoxically, modern day swingers are, in many ways, exploring something that has been practiced for centuries. By bringing variety and adventure into their sex lives, they are inviting new energy and vitality. The way that people approach this activity, however, can make all the difference. If it is done without awareness and respect it can, from an energetic point of view, cause more harm than good.

Those who prepare themselves consciously and have sexual practices based on good communication, awareness, mutual respect and sexual energy management techniques can find themselves in the company of sacred sex adepts who have practiced this way for millennia. Despite the prevalent sex-negative conditioning in our society, we are seeing increasing interest in the creation of places and events where we can learn about, practice and experience the benefits of these age old techniques.

Questions you can ask yourself and each other

+ What does our sexual relationship look like?
+ How are we investing in our sexual relationship?
+ Do I know what my partner's needs and fantasies are?
+ Do I dare express my fantasies and desires? If yes, do I do it?
  If no, what would I need to be able to express them?
+ How do we handle our mutual needs and desires?
+ Which of my boundaries would I want to stretch if I had the chance?
+ How do I handle my partner's boundaries?

Tips if you are considering a swinger's lifestyle

+ Ensure that you have a solid and stable relationship with open and honest communication. Work on the success factors for a sustainable relationship.
+ Talk ahead of time about your wishes and expectations.
+ Take your time. Consider visiting a club and simply observing before you do decide to do anything yourselves.
+ Set your boundaries and take each other's boundaries seriously. Safety is essential both while swinging, and for the sustainability of your relationship.
+ Practice safe sex and use condoms. If you use alcohol and/or recreational drugs: do it with moderation! If you're not used to using alcohol and/or drugs, now is not the time to experiment with them.
+ Release any expectations that you might have, and enjoy the present.
+ Keep contact with your partner and consider agreeing on a stop word.
+ Sexual stimulation can be addictive. There is a risk that you can unintentionally cross your boundaries as you continue to look to experience new "sexual kicks." Keep your private sexual relationship with your partner alive, and continue to enjoy the intimacy and communication that you two have together.

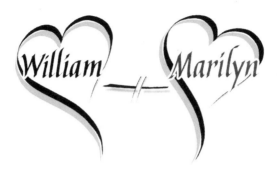

Loving Release:
When Paths Diverge —
Marilyn and William

You've been together for thirty years, and the children have started to leave home. A few years ago, your partner announced that he is polyamorous and told you that he wanted to make room for this in his life. You, on the other hand, are monogamous. Your partner has had a complementary relationship for a couple of years now and this is not something you are comfortable with. Together, you've tried to make your relationship work so that everyone can be happy, but without much success. The difficulty continues and sometimes the emotions run high. Slowly you're both running out of energy for your relationship and this is affecting not only each other but your whole family. What now?

Marilyn and William are working through this problem.

Marilyn (fifty-four) and William (fifty-one) have been married for twenty-seven years and have three children. Eight years ago, William had a secret affair with another woman. Marilyn was devastated when she found out about it, and was so relieved when William finally ended it to save their marriage. This was a dark period in Marilyn's life, and quite frankly she would rather forget about it. For William, it had been an experience with two sides: the energy and joy he felt with his new lover, and the confusion and guilt he felt when he thought about his wife and their marriage.

A few years ago, William read an article about polyamory. Somewhere inside he had always known that he could love more than one woman at once. He had often been attracted to other women or fallen in love. The article gave him the impetus to find out more about this. Eventually, William found an online forum for people who self-identify as polyamorous. This was such a relief for him as he realized that he was not the only who felt and thought the way he did. Through the forum, he began conversing with Elisabeth (forty-four). They started e-mailing each other privately soon after. Elisabeth had encouraged William to go and talk to Marilyn about the fact that he felt sure that he was polyamorous. Although William found this a very difficult thing to do, he bit the bullet and spoke to Marilyn about it. This was a painful and upsetting conversation for Marilyn. She had the feeling that she was being pulled into something that she had not asked for. She was not at all certain that she wanted anything to do with polyamory or William's exploration of it.

During this initial conversation, William told Marilyn that he no longer wanted to suppress and deny this part of his identity. He wanted to explore what being polyamorous meant for him. He wanted to make room in his life for his feelings for other women. He also wanted to meet Elisabeth in person. They'd been e-mailing for a while and lately had spoken to each other on the phone. It was clear that there was something happening between the two of them. William did not want to do anything behind Marilyn's back ever again. Since he knew the damaging consequences of lying and cheating, William preferred to be open and honest from now on. Marilyn appreciated that very much. She saw that it was difficult for William and that he was trying to be fair to both of them. Some part of her wanted to be able to allow him this freedom to love other women. She finally told William that she felt OK with him meeting with Elisabeth.

William and Elisabeth soon realized that they had fallen in love with each other and wanted to meet on a regular basis. Marilyn was hesitant, but she also wanted to give William the space to be himself. Anyway, who was she to hold him back? Above all she felt that if she wanted to stay in a relationship with William, she had to let him see Elisabeth. She loves William, and as a family and as a couple they are a great team. She didn't want to lose him.

As William's relationship with Elisabeth developed, so too did William's ability to state clearly what he wanted in his life. Marilyn began to feel that there was no stopping him. She couldn't change the fact that he was in love with someone else and, although painful, she had accepted it. For 18 months they worked on making sure that their emotional interactions were positive ones. They have succeeded, although it has been a difficult process.

The main problem they are facing is that Marilyn is very jealous. She finds it very upsetting when William sits at the computer chatting and e-mailing with Elisabeth. It feels like he is completely inaccessible to her when he does that. Whenever William has a date with Elisabeth, Marilyn finds herself worked up about it a few days beforehand; and if William stays the night with Elisabeth, Marilyn sleeps badly. It always takes a few days after William comes home before Marilyn allows herself to be intimate with him again. Elisabeth comes by the house sometimes as well. William is helping Elisabeth to write promotional text for charities. Elisabeth wants to set up her own foundation, and William is supporting her endeavor. Marilyn likes Elisabeth and thinks that she is a lovely, friendly and fun woman. This of course makes the whole situation even more difficult.

When William told Marilyn a few weeks ago that he wanted to go on holiday with Elisabeth it was simply too much for Marilyn. She has the feeling that she is constantly stretching her boundaries and that the process never seems to end. She couldn't bear the thought of William and Elisabeth going on holiday together. What would she tell her friends and family? Almost none of them knew of William's complementary relationship. The tension at home became almost unbearable and their son, the only one of their children that still lived with them, started to stay at his girlfriend's house to escape the screaming matches between William and Marilyn. Marilyn was the one who finally decided to set up an introductory session with Leonie to see if she could help.

Coming out as polyamorous

Many people who discover the existence of polyamory experience a Eureka! moment. Feelings that we've had for a while are suddenly acknowledged as real and we feel that our desires all of a sudden have a right to exist. We no longer need to suppress or deny this part of ourselves. "This is how I work, this is what I have experienced in my life. My feelings are normal and there are other people just like me!" Feelings resulting from affirmations such as these can provide an enormous energy boost. Weight falls from our shoulders and sometimes we even feel like shouting from the rooftops, and we instantly want to start doing something with our new self-identification. This can be a real problem if we are already in a relationship with someone who is monogamous, who does not feel polyamorous themselves, and who is not at all happy with our newly found sense of identity. This dual-existence, for example: feeling polyamorous but living in a monogamous relationship, can lead to internal struggles and external conflicts. We ask ourselves "Should I give in to my polyamorous feelings or not?" In the meantime, the pull to connect to our core being, and our desires to live lives based on who we truly are, often continue to increase. We feel that we want to explore ways of being authentic without being unfaithful to our partners. Many polyamorous people that are in this phase have a tendency to become fully absorbed in their individual process of development. We research as much as we can and we try to find people who understand us. Sometimes, when we finally tell our partners we are polyamorous we are, in terms of information and general knowledge, way ahead of them. For our partners, the news that we self-identify as polyamorous can often feel like a complete, and often rather unpleasant, shock. For someone who is monogamous — that is someone who is committed to feel love for one person at a time and who desires a relationship with just one partner — the notion of polyamory completely opposes their relationship paradigm.

Shortly after William and Marilyn arrived at my practice, I asked them to each tell their side of the story, with no interruptions from the other partner. Marilyn told her story first. As she spoke I noticed that it was very difficult for the two of them not to interrupt each other. William wanted very much to highlight his side of the story even as Marilyn spoke, and had a tendency to take over the conversation if left unchecked. His behavior made it clear that he tended to steer the relationship. It turns out that Marilyn sometimes feels that she doesn't have enough space or opportunity to find out what she actually wants in the relationship. She has the feeling that she has been forced into the open relationship that she is now in, even though she knows that she has agreed to it. When she married William she had definitely not chosen to be in an open relationship. She married him because she loved him and wanted to grow old with him. She still wants that, which is why she is doing everything in her power to get her negative feelings under control and to find a way to continue to be committed to the relationship in some form. She wants to give William space and freedom, but she finds it incredibly difficult and painful to do so. Her jealousy is getting the better of her to the extent that she is slowly becoming exhausted by it.

The whole situation with William's polyamory has meant that William and Marilyn have spoken a great deal with each other during the last few years. Their communication has improved and their intimate relationship has benefited as well. Marilyn sees these as positive developments and is happy with the way they have grown from their experience. But, she asks herself whether the relationship with Elisabeth is necessary for this to have happened. Couldn't they have done this without her? Marilyn wonders if their own relationship had been better, would William have needed the relationship with Elisabeth at all? Marilyn has the feeling that she is not good enough as a woman. No matter how often William tells her that he loves her for who is she is, her inner critic tells her that if only she had a bit more to her, William would be satisfied with her alone.

This sense of inadequacy is reinforced every time William spends the night at Elisabeth's. William often comes home from Elisabeth's place and wants to make love with Marilyn to show her that he still loves her; but Marilyn is simply not up for it and has a tendency to withdraw instead. She just can't understand how he could want to be intimate with her when he has just been with another woman, and yet he clearly does. This adds to her feeling of not being good enough for William. She feels stuck in a vicious circle, since the more William wants to see Elisabeth, the more she retreats and is less willing to meet his desires for intimacy. Marilyn's greatest fear is that Elisabeth will ultimately pull William towards her and that Marilyn will lose him completely. Why would he stay with a woman that is always jealous and wants to have sex less and less?

Marilyn has tried everything she knows to keep her jealousy in check, but with little success. In the beginning, she would simply stay at home when William was away, but she noticed that she didn't do much else than worry and cry. So she tried to distract herself. Sometimes she visited friends, but because she was always thinking of William, she wasn't fully present, and so she felt like she wasn't being fair to her friends. Nowadays, she often goes to the cinema when William is at Elisabeth's. At least her attention is on something else then, and if she does start to think about William she isn't bothering anyone else with it. Yet, she doesn't really enjoy using William and Elisabeth's trysts as an excuse to see films, and now something that she used to enjoy feels tainted too. Marilyn really only wants one thing: to get rid of her jealousy. She has heard of "compersion" (empathetic joy when a partner experiences happiness with someone else) but that is not something she feels yet. However, she has reached the point that she can accept William and Elisabeth hugging each other in her presence. Marilyn admits Elisabeth is definitely a woman that one could love.

William's experience is totally different. He's happy that he can be open and honest with Marilyn and that they have progressed so far in their relationship. It hurts him deeply to see that Marilyn is in such pain, but he feels that he can no longer be untrue to himself and that he can't, and won't, deny his feelings for Elisabeth. He also believes that even if he hadn't met Elisabeth, he would have fallen in love with someone else eventually. William no longer wants to deny his polyamorous inclinations. He feels much lighter for having identified his feelings, and feels so much more honest with himself. He mentioned that his chronic stiff-neck problems have disappeared since discovering his polyamorous identity and establishing his complementary relationship with Elisabeth.

William admitted that his relationship with Marilyn has required a lot of attention lately as it is changing. He feels that Marilyn has always been very dependent on him and that she is happy with that and would like to keep it that way. However, as far as he is concerned they've now moved into a new phase in their relationship. He's gone through a great deal of personal development and growth since meeting Elisabeth and it is of course having an impact on his relationship with Marilyn as well. Marilyn and he have been talking much more with each other and he thinks their communication has improved markedly, though he realized that lately he is beginning to get a bit impatient. He's doing his best to allow Marilyn to set the pace but he has the feeling that if it were up to her he would never see Elisabeth again, and consequently all growth in his relationship with Marilyn would stop. On top of that, no matter what he does, it's never good enough. If he chooses to see Elisabeth, he hurts Marilyn. If he chooses not to see Elisabeth, he hurts himself. It seems like a no-win situation.

Trying to find ways to deal with the situation with both women is beginning to get to William. He feels impatient, and sometimes he can no longer be bothered to take Marilyn into account. The fact that he is choosing to do what he wants to do leaves him with tremendous feelings of guilt the minute he realizes what he is doing. The arguments that occur when he does lose patience are intense at times and he sometimes succumbs to sharp outbursts of anger, which is uncharacteristic and quite unsettling. He feels that it would help if Marilyn could learn to handle her jealousy a bit better. It would make life easier for everyone and above all keep the atmosphere at home more relaxed. He has the feeling that there is no way they can go another eighteen months with the situation as it is now. He absolutely does not want to lose Marilyn though. She is his wife, his friend, the mother of his children and his life partner. He thinks that it must be possible to find a solution. His trust in their love for each other is enormous.

The mono-poly relationship

We might call a relationship between someone who is "mono-amorous" and someone who is "poly-amorous," a "mono-poly relationship."

This is not one of the easiest pairings. It is a relationship form that often asks a lot of both partners since they each have very different views of what a relationship is. There are monos who do manage to find a relationship form that can accommodate these paradigm conflicts, however to thrive as a mono in an open relationship requires a certain amount of independence and autonomy. It helps if we are comfortable with ourselves and are not dependent on our partners for our own happiness and amusement. A good dose of flexibility and the ability to see things from other people's points of view are also helpful; and self-compassion and empathy for our partners are indispensable. On top of this, it is important that we foster good connections with our partners. In addition to love and emotional support, it is helpful to find other interests that bring us together.

Different people find different solutions to the mono-poly conundrum. Sometimes a poly decides not to express his or her polyamorous side and instead engages in a monogamous relationship. He or she may feel love for someone other than his or her partner, but would never have an intimate or sexual relationship outside the committed relationship. The most that the committed relationship can accommodate is a close friendship with the third person within clearly set boundaries. In such cases, the poly adjusts his or her desire to express love for more than one person to the needs of the mono who wants a monogamous relationship.

It also happens that monogamous boundaries are stretched to include a limited sexual relationship outside the committed partnership, or that the boundaries are set so that a complementary relationship can include cuddling and kissing. Other monos give their polyamorous partners more freedom and try to find their own ways to deal with jealousy. Yet others choose to have a "triad" in a "V" form, where the polyamorous partner acts as the "pivot." Even in this case, the mono may need to work on managing his or her jealousy issues. Sometime a mono-poly relationship simply ceases to exist when the mono person hears that his or her partner is in love with someone else and wants to make room in his or her relationship for this. For some monos, there are no acceptable mono-poly solutions as far as they are concerned.

Mono-poly situations are complex and, as such, benefit from well-considered decisions. This includes giving everyone concerned all the time and space needed to find out what really works and not to simply make decisions based on strong initial emotions. Some couples take years to come to a place of balance in their new relationship forms. Others finally come to the conclusion that they will never be happy in a mono-poly relationship. It is important to take time to make the decision, even if it takes years.

Many polyamorous people have a tendency to move much too quickly when trying to find ways to incorporate polyamory into their existing monogamous relationships. This is especially true when they are in love and full of NRE (New Relationship Energy). Many times, monos find it difficult to acknowledge and really accept that their partners are polyamorous. They find it incomprehensible that their partners can love them *and* someone else at the same time, much less want to express it in some fashion. Their pictures of relationships as twosomes fall to pieces when their partners make poly revelations. This change can destroy confidence and expectations for their relationships. This is very difficult for many monos. It's not surprising then that many monos in mono-poly relationships maintain a prolonged state of denial regarding their partners' poly tendencies. Indeed, it's not easy to move at the same pace.

Marilyn felt that William moved much too quickly when his new love appeared on the scene. He had already started a new, complementary relationship with Elisabeth while Marilyn had barely gotten used to the idea that her husband is polyamorous. In reality, she didn't really want to know about his decision to identify as polyamorous. Somewhere deep inside, she thought that the only reason William was making such a claim was that their own relationship wasn't good enough for him. She also felt that if she did not accept Elisabeth in William's life, she would lose him sooner or later, as he had made it abundantly clear that he did not want to return to a monogamous relationship. Marilyn felt like she had been put into a no-win situation and that she was the victim. Even though she had agreed to William and Elisabeth's first meeting, in her heart she had screamed in protest.

During the following session we played *The Relationship Game*. This highlighted the facts that William and Marilyn have a strong emotional bond and that they share a great deal. This session made their connections to each other clearer and as a result they realized that it was worth carrying on with the process of finding a solution. The "Behavior Cards" that they chose helped them to see that Marilyn finds it difficult to share her feelings with other people and to voice what her needs are. As we examined Marilyn's behavior more closely, it became apparent that she often follows along rather than alerting others to the fact that she is uncomfortable. I challenged Marilyn to stand up more for herself and to be more upfront with her feelings. During this coaching session I focused my attention primarily on Marilyn. As we progressed, William began to realize that the difference between their respective speeds of change was much greater than he had initially thought. William was constantly asking Marilyn to stretch her boundaries, which resulted in Marilyn often feeling that she scarcely had any time to consider what she could actually cope with. Marilyn often agrees with William simply because she does not want to lose him.

I asked Marilyn what she would need to be able to know where her boundaries and limits are. She said that what she really needed was a bit of peace and quiet to be able think and to feel — a space of internal calmness. The primary source of Marilyn's internal chaos and constant worry were the nights that William spent with Elisabeth and the recurring pain that occurred afterwards. This was difficult for William to hear.

He had the feeling that he had to constantly hold back on his contact with Elisabeth. If it was up to him he'd rather spend more, not less, time with Elisabeth but that was not possible as things stood. At this point Marilyn asked William if he would put his relationship with Elisabeth temporarily on hold. William felt like he was now the one being given an ultimatum. He was afraid that if he acquiesced in her request, Marilyn would feel like she won and that everything would go back to the way it had been.

I asked William what would be necessary for him to be able to trust that this would be a good decision for the sake of his relationship with Marilyn. William said that he would need to know that it was a temporary decision. He would want to know that Marilyn would make a serious effort to do something about her jealousy. After a long discussion they made a three month agreement. This was a terribly long time for William but he understood that Marilyn needed this. They compromised on the terms of their agreement: William would only contact Elisabeth from home via e-mail, but not telephone. William would see Elisabeth in person no more than once a month and would not stay overnight at her house. William and Elisabeth could kiss and cuddle when they did meet, but they would refrain from sex. William and Marilyn would set aside one evening a week to talk. Marilyn would have some individual coaching sessions to work on her jealousy. She would tell William what happened during these sessions. We all agreed that this would happen on a basis of complete openness and transparency with each other.

Looking into the mirror

Every relationship that we engage in offers us opportunities to look in the mirror: to reflect upon our own behavior and to look at our feelings. Relationships usually give us chances to grow, as they often highlight our imperfections. In open or polyamorous relationships, this process can be intensified and it is usually not possible to avoid self-reflection at all. There are simply more partners to learn from and often there is, metaphorically, nowhere to hide. Unfortunately, the greater the number of people involved, the more chances there are for jealousy to take hold. The real question when this starts to happen is, do we really want to look in the mirror? Not everyone is willing to do this, especially when it comes to jealousy. For many people, analyzing jealousy is simply too much to handle. They see huge mountains of unresolved issues in front of them and feel that there is no way to work their way through. They hope instead to find ways around examining their worries or to simply escape.

Escape strategies

There are a number of ways to try to avoid dealing with pain in a situation. Experience has shown that in the long term, none of them ultimately work. It can be very useful to be aware of these tactics, though, as escaping is a human way of handling difficult situations, and it's easy enough to find ourselves trying. Roughly speaking there are nine different escape strategies:

1. **ESCAPE INTO THE PAST.** We constantly think back to the time when everything was better, when it seems like there were clear boundaries and clarity about the future. We had such a good time then, if only it could be that way again. We hope that there is still a chance that our partners will change when they see what a hard time we are having, and that everything will go back to the way it was.

2. **ESCAPE INTO UNREALISTIC HOPES FOR THE FUTURE.** We believe that when a bit of time has passed things will surely go better. Maybe our partners' new love will tire of being the third person and leave, and then we'll have our partners back all for ourselves again.

3. **BLAME THE OTHER PERSON.** There's nothing wrong with us. If our partners would only realize the difficulty they are causing they would put a stop to all the nonsense. If our partners really loved us they wouldn't do this to us. It's our partner's fault and anyway they are expecting the impossible of us.

4. **ESCAPE INTO PASSIVITY.** Oh, what's the point anyway? No matter what we attempt, it's doomed to failure. How many relationships like this work anyway? Probably not many. So why bother with this or anything for that matter? We move into passivity and retreat from the situation. We say less and less, and our partners despair more as a result.

5. **ESCAPE INTO NEGATIVE BELIEFS ABOUT OURSELVES.** Look at us — we're useless! We're not good enough, so who would love us anyway? If we were good enough for our partners, no one else would be needed. Anyway, we're ugly and unattractive, right? We focus our attention on our perceived negative aspects and beat ourselves up when something unpleasant happens. Our negative beliefs ensure that we can see no options for moving forward, and we become despondent and depressed.

6. **TAKE REFUGE IN "PEOPLE-PLEASER" BEHAVIOR.** If we only do our very best, maybe our partners will love us so much that they won't need anyone else. In order to feel good about ourselves, we look to our partners for praise and affirmations. We become so dependent on these that we start to change our behavior in order to fulfill his or her requests or demands and end up being less true to ourselves.

7. **ESCAPE INTO FALSE INDEPENDENCE.** Everything's fine with us. No, there's nothing bothering us, why do you ask? Life is grand and everything is under control. We focus on other things and let everyone know that we can manage all by ourselves. Any assistance offered is kindly but firmly refused.

8. **ESCAPE INTO HUMOR.** If things get difficult we always joke about it so that we can both laugh. We avoid serious discussions with a wise-crack or two. We try to find something funny in every situation and constantly use humor as an excuse.

9. **ESCAPE INTO SUBSTANCE ABUSE OR COMPULSIVE BEHAVIOR.** We drink too much alcohol, use mind-altering drugs or engage in behavior such as compulsive gambling or constantly playing computer games to flee from reality. Our feelings and negative thoughts are anesthetized or suppressed.

Acknowledging reality

All of the above ways of reacting and escaping are focused on alleviating the pain that has been created by a new dimension in our relationships. When we escape, we place the blame for our situations on someone or something else. We thereby rob ourselves of the possibility to stand in our power and to invest in ourselves and, by extension, our relationships. The only way to get clear about a plan for the future, whatever it may be, is in fact to deal with the pain. It is only when we can look reality square in the face that we can bid the relationship-that-was farewell. If we release our resistance to letting go, we will notice that we suddenly gain the space to feel and to consider how we would like to deal with our new situations. When we acknowledge and accept reality, we are free to investigate all the possibilities as well as the impossibilities, and make well-considered decisions.

The first step we took in helping Marilyn come to grips with her jealousy — and to become fully present and aware of the reality of her situation — was to help her to improve her self-image. Using the *Core Qualities Game* from Daniel Ofman, we highlighted the qualities that make Marilyn a unique individual. Marilyn discovered that she had more virtues than she thought she did. Until now, she tended toward only recognizing her negative qualities, such as the fact that she allowed people to override her wishes too often. Marilyn started to build a more positive picture of herself when she recognized her favorable qualities that corresponded with each perceived negativity, such as her caring demeanor and her ability to empathize. I asked her to do some homework and to ask people she knew to give her feedback about herself; and this turned out to be a positive experience. She received many friendly and well-meant responses and tips from people who are close to her.

I subsequently helped Marilyn to discover more about her blind spots and how to deal with them. She realized that she wants to stand up more for herself and set her boundaries better. She also learned that it is better to say what's bothering her sooner rather than later. In that way she can demonstrate her self-respect. She also discovered that she can use her sense of humor to make situations a bit lighter and more bearable.

During the subsequent sessions we started to work directly on her jealousy. We did this using a guided meditation. This was a tough session for Marilyn, with many tears. She uncovered a whole list of negative thoughts with corresponding fears. She is convinced that Elisabeth is better in bed than she is and that Elisabeth gives William what he needs: a warm woman that loves to cuddle and have sex. She also holds onto the idea that she has nothing to say about the form her relationship with William has taken, and that he decides on most issues based on what he wants: room for Elisabeth in his life. Marilyn is afraid that she is not good enough to exist; afraid of not being heard; fears being left in the lurch and losing her place in life; and fears she is not unique and is therefore easily replaceable.

Marilyn found it difficult to see this list laid out so clearly. She was very resistant to the thought of starting to look at her thoughts and fears in terms of their origination. Despite this, Marilyn did acknowledge, once she saw it, that she has a tendency to create negative beliefs about herself. She also understands that she often employs the people-pleaser escape strategy as she is forever giving in to William's wishes. Her most commonly used escape tendencies, however, are to take refuge in the past and to have unrealistic expectations.

We took a short trip to the past to have a look at where her fears come from. This was not easy for Marilyn as she did not like to talk about her childhood. It was clear to her though that her people-pleaser behavior was something that she brought with her from her youth. She had a dominating and perfectionist father whose wishes were commands, and a subservient mother who liked to keep father happy. By being nice to others, Marilyn had earned the appreciation from her mother that she had so longed for. Her father never gave Marilyn compliments and set his expectations for her very high with the result that she never felt good enough. He often screamed at her and her sisters and told them that they were all the same. They shouldn't whine so much, and should shut up and stop being so stupid. If Marilyn ever protested, she was told to be quiet, and sometimes Marilyn's father physically chastised her. As a result, Marilyn learned to keep things to herself at an early age.

I suggested to Marilyn that we could schedule a separate session where, with the help of a visualization, we would go back to her youth. She could then acknowledge her pain and put some events into their correct places as a way of healing the trauma. Hesitantly, she agreed. Two weeks later, though, Marilyn told me that after careful consideration, she decided that she really didn't feel like going back and looking at the past as a way of dealing with what was happening. She had enough problems in the present and she wanted to use the relative calm that she had with William, now that he was not having sex with Elisabeth, to look towards the future. Lately, she had been asking herself whether it would not be better if she and William should go their own separate ways. As a result of all the conversations, she realized that she was tired of fighting. On the other hand, she didn't want to simply give up on the relationship. She felt she was in a bind and asked me if I knew of a way to allow her to look at her life in a different way.

The seven years writing exercise

I gave her the "seven years writing" exercise. This is a practical way for Marilyn to look back at her life as if it was a book. The exercise entails dividing her life into periods of seven years. Each one of these periods then becomes a chapter with its own title, and this title reflects the essence of that particular period. Sometimes, it's helpful to write down a few key words for each period as well. It is important to carefully contemplate and aptly title each period. The process continues until the current period of life is reached.

As we created the drawing, Marilyn and I looked back at her life from her birth until the present. She found it difficult to come up with titles herself so we talked about each chapter and then summarized. This made it easier for Marilyn to come up with titles that matched her feelings. We wrote the headings on a whiteboard, and Marilyn saw an overview of her life. First, she saw how influential her youth was on her adult life. It also became very clear that the years when her children were young had been the happiest years of her life. She had been able to put her worries to one side and concentrate on creating a family with William. This gave her life both structure and meaning. In her current period of forty-nine — fifty-six, life had been turned totally upside down. She joked that the title of this period should be "Upside Down." I challenged her to do just that. She took the pen, turned the entire whiteboard upside down and wrote the title. When she looked at the whiteboard in its original position she started to cry. "That's exactly what it is. I no longer want to feel like my life is standing on its head." We stopped then and considered what exactly "standing on its head" meant for her. As a result, it became clear that an open relationship simply does not suit Marilyn. She had been trying to survive by attempting to overcome her awkward position. She felt like she was a turtle that was on its back with its legs thrashing and could no longer move. She wanted to get back to living, not simply surviving.

I asked her to consider how she would like to fill in the following periods of her life. How would she like the story of her life to continue? What would she like her grandchildren to read about her life if they found her life story? What would the story look like if she simply continued to wait and see what happened, as she had done until now? How could she decide for herself which way her life was going to go? What would the title of the following chapter be if she no longer wanted her life to be upside down? What would the title of the next chapter be if she carried on in her relationship with William?

We looked at two possibilities, life with William and life without him. Marilyn realized that if she ended the relationship there would be a period of mourning and goodbyes, but that she would free up possibilities to move her life in new directions. The title in such a case would be "Taking Leave and Beginning Again." If she stayed with William, it would continue to be an upside down life and the title would be "Continuing Pain." But she did not want that any longer. This observation made Marilyn sad, but also brought clarity and a sense of relief. She told me that she wanted to continue with the exercise at home and wanted to talk to William about it. Our next session would include the three of us.

Acknowledging that we are different from each other

It takes courage to take a good hard look at reality, especially if two people love each other very much, are in a long-term relationship and have built up a long common past together. However, sometimes loving each other very much is not enough to be able to stay together. If each person's respective relationship requirements and wishes start to diverge so much that there is no agreeable relationship structure, then it can be better to part ways. Choosing to stay together as a mono-poly couple means that both partners need to be prepared, out of love for each other, to sacrifice a part of their own needs. This is certainly the case in the beginning of a changed relationship. Poly people need to take into account the feelings of their mono partners and therefore accept that they might not be able to develop their poly relationships in the speed and fashion that they would like. They will also need to be prepared to be constantly reminded that their choices can be painful for their partners, no matter how illogical that may seem. The knowledge that they are hurting their partners will unavoidably lead to them feeling pain themselves, especially if they love their partners very much. They may have to be prepared, then, to offer their mono partners support and acknowledgement for their pain.

Mono people will, on the other hand, need courage to dare to acknowledge that their poly partners view their relationship forms differently. Mono people will need to be prepared to deal with the inevitable issues that will arise. In addition, mono people will need to acknowledge their poly partners' pain, as they constantly try to accommodate their mono partners' feelings and as a result may well be suppressing their own needs concerning other relationships.

Although many people do manage to make mono-poly relationships work by using a great deal of compassion and empathy, many don't. Not everyone is prepared to make the sacrifices and effort required, even if many of the issues are resolved over time. The pain that a mono-poly relationship can create can be so overwhelming that both parties realize that it is better for both of them to begin to build up more authentic, separate lives.

Marilyn spoke with William at length about the seven-years exercise. The three month period of pause between William and Elisabeth together with the seven years exercise had made it clear to Marilyn that she wants to stop making room in their relationship for William to see Elisabeth, or any other women for that matter. She did not want to be constantly confronted with the pain this caused her. She asked William whether he was prepared to return to a monogamous marriage.

The truth was that, during the last couple of years, William had often asked himself that very same question. He had long ago ascertained that he did not want to return to a monogamous relationship, even if Marilyn couldn't deal with it. For the first time in his life, he feels liberated and true to himself. And that is good for him. "You can't stuff a butterfly back into the cocoon" declared William. "It has grown and gone through metamorphosis and that's that. If you try to put it back into the cocoon it will suffocate and die." William feels like he's been adapting to Marilyn's marital needs for years. He had often suppressed and denied his feelings for other women on Marilyn's account and it had created physical symptoms of stress. He never wants to do that again. He knows that a monogamous lifestyle does not suit him, and when he pretends to be a monogamous person, he denies his true identity. He is so happy to finally be clear about this. His relationship with Elisabeth has shown him that each relationship gives him an opportunity to grow and practice self-reflection. It is a way for him to get to know himself better and a way to find inner wholeness. Elisabeth is so different from Marilyn, and he enjoys that. For him one is no better than the other, he loves both of them. Now Marilyn is (as he sees it) forcing him to make a choice, and he understands that they will need to end their marriage. As he contemplates this, he feels how much he loves her and how painful it will be to release her, even if this is for the sake of being true to himself. He has no idea how to deal with his grief and sorrow and a feeling of despair overcomes him.

Parting ways

The decision to end a relationship and to each go our separate way is often accompanied by intense and often varying feelings: disbelief, denial, powerlessness, sadness and anger take turns. Given all the good we have had together, why can't we carry on? We feel frustrated since we've tried so hard to save our relationships, and at the end of the day it still breaks down. We feel the limits of our abilities. And we feel the sorrow of the coming goodbyes. It can even feel like the ground is disappearing from under our feet as all the plans that we've had for the future are suddenly no more. Feelings of emptiness and loneliness can also play a part. It's not only our partners we are saying good-bye to, it's also a good-bye to a family structure as we knew it, to an economic unit, and to a social unit. Our social network can react in different ways. Sometimes we get support from a direction we had never imagined, other times we feel abandoned as friends take sides. Also, the actual divorce and moving out of the house has repercussions that need to be dealt with. Splitting up means there is a long period where a great deal occurs. It is therefore important to take it step by step. This is a process where grieving plays an important part.

Taking farewell consciously

Ending a relationship and saying good bye to someone in a conscious and aware fashion is not something that our culture is used to. We can leave our jobs, and often parties or celebrations are given to honor us — complete with speeches and acclaim from our colleagues. Sometimes, our neighbors organize farewell parties when we move out of town. If we are going to get married we consciously say goodbye to our single lives with stag or hen parties. If someone dies we have many rituals that allow us to display and share our grief with others. But consciously saying goodbye to a relationship is not something we often do. Still, it can be beneficial to take the time to say goodbye to an intimate relationship and possibly even celebrate the event with a parting ritual.

Parting rituals

A parting ritual is a time to pause at the passage between one phase of life and another. By choosing to grieve together we can also work through our sorrow better. What about taking time together to look back at all the periods when we loved, laughed, enjoyed, argued and cared for each other? We can choose to make conscious, loving farewells to each other. There is nothing wrong with grieving for a relationship as it was, or grieving for the loss of our common futures as our perceived senses of security disappears. By allowing ourselves to acknowledge and experience the feelings and emotions that parting brings forth, we can acknowledge our losses as well as our freed possibilities. We can say goodbye to the connections that are no longer healthy, and release them. We can also say goodbye to certain phases of our lives. We leave the old behind. By doing this consciously we create room for new things, and hasten our healing.

There are various rituals we can use to consciously say goodbye to a relationship. We can buy a big bouquet of flowers and hang a little card on each flower with a text or a symbol that stands for a certain period of our lives. When the flowers have finished blooming, we can bury them or burn the cards. Through the cards, we can express appreciation for what the relationship has brought us, and then let go. Or, we can paint a picture for each other and express visually the time we have spent together in relationship. We can create a collage of old photographs from our time together. We can create (or ask an artist or artistic friend to create) a sculptural piece out of items that have significance to both of us. We can write a letter to each other where we say goodbye to our relationship as it was, read the letters to each other and then ceremoniously let the letters go.

If we are not in a state to carry out any sort of ritual at the time of our parting, we can always do it later when we have more energy, or when the worst grief and sorrow has passed. During this period of mourning, we can go for a walk together and pick up a stone, and speak aloud all of our thoughts and pain and misery to this stone, and then throw it into a river or stream. Let the earth recycle our grief.

Goodbye rituals are also a way to, in a dignified and gentle fashion, acknowledge and accept that there may be pain that has either caused, or has been caused by, the ending of relationships. This can be an important step in moving forward and releasing that pain. If the pain is so great that it is not possible to organize rituals, or if we simply wish not to do this, it can also help to have a friend participate in some sort of parting ceremony with us instead. It's not so important how we do it, but it can be a great help to take the time to bid farewell and move forward with awareness.

Out with the old, in with the new
—OLD ENGLISH EXPRESSION

William and Marilyn took the time to grieve about the loss of their intimate relationship and their shared family life. First they did this together by writing each other a letter. They then went for a walk on the beach and read sections of their letters to each other. All the periods of their life together were mentioned: when they got to know each other, their wedding, the birth of their children, their holidays together, and the last years together. When they finished reading their letters to each other they tied them to a stone and threw the stone into the sea. They walked back in silence, each lost in his or her own thoughts. In the meantime, it started to rain. They felt as though the wind and the rain washed their thoughts and emotions clean.

It was only after William and Marilyn had taken farewell of their marriage that they felt that the time was right to speak to their children of it. The children were shocked. Apart from the son that was living at home, they had little exposure to the ups and down of the relationship between their parents. Not all the children reacted positively. There were a number of discussions between the parents and the children. For William and Marilyn it was clear: this was an issue between the two of them only. They would always be there for their children and they would always be their parents. Just because they were divorcing did not mean that they would disappear out of each other's lives. In fact, it took William nine months to find a new place to live.

During this period Marilyn continued her coaching sessions for support in her emotional process and in setting up a new life for herself. A lot of attention went into her feelings of loneliness. She learned how to pay more attention to herself and less to William, who she felt dependent on, and her situation slowly improved.

When William finally moved into his new flat, he and Marilyn entered a new separation phase, saying goodbye to their life together. Marilyn and William indicated to the children that it would be nice if they would also take part in a good-bye ceremony. Two of three agreed to this, the third wanted nothing to do with it. Together they had a final Sunday at home. William cooked a wonderful meal and Marilyn had taken time during the last few weeks to gather up all the family pictures and put them in albums. In this way they took the time to stop and appreciate their life as a family.

When William left, Marilyn consciously decided to create distance between them. She wanted to get in touch with herself and to find out what part of her self-image was indeed hers, what was William's and what was both of theirs. William found it very upsetting that Marilyn was not in touch for a time, but he understood. They agreed that Marilyn would reestablish contact when she felt the time was right. After a few months, Marilyn called William and they met and talked. There were feelings of sadness, but also happiness and thankfulness that they could share so much with each other. They felt their connection would always be there and they both felt, despite the pain associated with the ending of their relationship, that they had made the right choice. They each looked forward to a future that was more congruent to their true selves, and at the same time found a way to keep their love for each other in their hearts.

CELEBRATING TRANSITIONS
IN THE NA CULTURE

The Na culture in China, also known as the Moso, manages the end of a relationship very differently than we do in the West. In the Na culture, the primary family unit is based around women; and relationships with men are purely based on love and affection. In other words, for the Na the end of a relationship is not the catastrophe that it is for women in cultures where many women tend to be dependent on men for their financial and day-to-day security. The Na way of starting and ending relationships is beautiful and touching in its clarity and simplicity. They simply sing to each other! When a relationship is beginning a couple might sing:

"You are the salt to my tea" (the Na put salt in their tea)
to indicate that romance was in the air.

When a Na relationship comes to an end, the song reflects the parting:

If there is no love
My heart will not feel
If there is no wind
The clouds above the mountain will not move
Since we are trees from two different mountains
Our branches will never reach each other
The water flows in the creek
But the creek will not bend for the water

Recently, when asked about their custom of "walking marriage" a Na man spoke of what he called the unrealistic view of marriage in other cultures. "The Na hold the search for true love higher than anything else" he explained. "That's why we keep our relationships open. It gives us the chance to keep looking for the perfect partner. We feel that other cultures are hypocritical when they expect true love the first time round.... The Na aren't obsessed with sex, it's just a natural part of things." When the end of a relationship is considered a normal part of life, as it is with Na, saying goodbye need not be the dramatic and traumatic event that it often is in the West.

Questions you can ask yourself

+ How do I deal with my dissatisfaction in my relationship?
+ How do I acknowledge my partner's different ways of seeing the world?
+ What basic psychological needs did I not have met as a child? What messages did I get from my parent(s)?
+ What survival strategies do I recognize from my childhood? How do they apply to my relationship?
+ How do I say goodbye to things that once were in my relationship but are now gone?

Tips for releasing lovingly

+ Dare to stand up for your feelings and to experience the associated feelings. They're allowed to be. Remember that you have feelings but your feelings do not define who you are.
+ Take time to grieve. Grieving does not happen in a day. It can take up to a year or more. As you go through each season, holiday, anniversary, there will be renewed memories and emotions that will take time to experience and work through.
+ Don't try to suppress your feelings, allow your tears to flow. Dare to allow yourself to be sad, even if the sadness seems overwhelming.
+ Find a parting ceremony or ritual that suits your relationship. Have the courage to fully engage with the ritual and its healing energy.
+ Look for support and consolation. Friends or family can help. You can also do this by being kind to yourself — for instance book a massage, take a retreat, enjoy a spa day, etc. A pet can provide consolation too.
+ Write down your sorrows and your joys. Start a journal or diary and end each day by noting something positive that you have valued during the day. It can be a small thing, like the color of a flower, the taste of a good cup of coffee; or it can be a grand thing like the laugh from someone you care about.
+ Dare to ask for help if you get stuck and can't manage on your own.

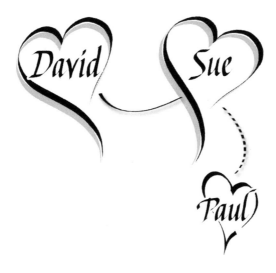

10

The End Of Sex, Or Maybe Not? — David and Sue

You've built a good relationship and have been together for years. There have been ups and downs over time but you've come through them, and you are stronger as a result. As a woman, you are in your prime and enjoy your family, your work, friends and holidays. The truth is, you've nothing to complain about — except your sex life. You're just fine but your partner is, as a result of a number of circumstances, no longer what he was. To be honest: you don't have sex with each other anymore and the chances of doing anything is about zero. It's becoming apparent that in all likelihood you will forgo sex entirely if you stay with your partner. But to leave each other on the basis of no sex seems crazy. So what can you do about it? Do you need to accept that you can forget about having an active sex life for the rest of your life?

David, thirty-nine, and Sue, thirty-seven, have been together for fifteen years and have an eleven-year-old daughter, Lucy. David is the customer-service manager for a large multinational company. Sue works in sales for an advertising agency. In many ways they are opposites. David is calm itself. He is always on top of things and provides the stable, emotional and practical basis for the household and the relationship. He enjoys working with computers and electronics and is very handy around the house. Sue, on the other hand, would much rather be out with friends. She is a lively, expressive woman that easily takes the initiative and enjoys entertaining and having fun. They complement each other perfectly.

David, however, had a health setback seven years ago. The well-balanced man who could always calm everyone during periods of stress and crisis had become increasingly withdrawn. He was no longer himself. Eventually, his doctor diagnosed severe depression. It appears that there is a history of depression in David's family. His father was continually depressed and his grandfather had committed suicide during a bout of depression. David had been referred to a psychiatrist who prescribed antidepressants and therapy. David finally recovered from the dark place he'd been in, but when he attempted to come off the antidepressants it did not go well. The psychiatrist advised David to continue taking the antidepressants and indicated that he would probably need to do this for the rest of his life. David was very upset when the doctor told him this as the antidepressants have a devastating effect on his sex drive. His depressive thoughts and feelings have indeed disappeared as a result of the medication, but so has his desire for sex. Sex has become a chore and is a disappointing experience for both David and Sue. During the last few years, David has switched medications hoping that things would improve but to no avail. Finally, David has decided that he would rather have a life that works without sex than a morose life that includes sex.

Sue is happy that peace and calm have returned to their home, and she enjoys more time and space for herself now that David is cheerful once again. Having a deeply depressed partner had been very difficult… yet she hasn't quite accepted the lack of sex in their otherwise good partnership.

One evening not long ago when she was out with a group of friends, the conversation turned to sex. It was really tough for Sue to be reminded that other women were having great sex — and that she wasn't. Sue felt like an outsider as she'd not had sex for years. She still cuddled with David but lively, passionate sex was simply no longer in the cards with him. One of her friends spoke of rediscovering sexual passion in a new relationship and joked "Yes ladies, life begins at forty!" A lump formed in Sue's throat, and her eyes welled with tears as she thought about her sex life ending before she even reached forty. One of her friends noticed this and the talk turned serious. As a result of their gentle and caring questions, Sue spoke of her situation and her feelings. Her friends were tremendously supportive and compassionate.

The talk with her girlfriends gave Sue serious food for thought. Did she really want to be celibate for the rest of her life? Yes, of course she could make do with self-pleasuring but that was just not the same thing as spending time with a man — touching each other's bodies and real sex with all that it entailed. In an effort to rekindle her sexual relationship with David, Sue began to mention her issues around her sex life, or the lack thereof, more often to David. The result was not what she had hoped for. Instead of provoking constructive discussion, the topic soon led to increased friction and irritation between them. In the meantime, Sue was so full of sexual desire that she caught herself fantasizing about seducing the cute guy who delivered parcels to their house. Of course you don't do such things! Anyway, she didn't want to cheat, she couldn't bear the thought of secrecy or of lying. How did other women in the same situation deal with this predicament? She couldn't be the only one with this problem! One evening, Sue found Leonie's web site, and convinced David that it might be worth talking with a professional about their situation. So, she gave Leonie a call.

The absence of a sexual relationship

There are countless couples who love each other dearly and yet have sexless relationships. Sometimes there are medical reasons, but it also happens that the sexual passion between the partners has simply disappeared over the years. They are often great couples that work well as a team and as parents, and they are satisfied with what they have built up together. If both partners are happy with their sex-free relationships then everything is fine. However, if one of the partners needs sex this can lead to problems. Sexual needs are very human and many people experience a lifelong need for sexual contact, eroticism and intimacy. Sex is a source of life energy and health. In fact, some research shows that women and men who enjoy sex tend to live longer than those who don't.

In sexless relationships, there are no straightforward ways for partners who need sex to satisfy their needs. After all, most of us are raised with the notion that we have sex with our partners and no one else. Sex is something intimate that we only share with our partners. Or is it?

One of the first things I did when David and Sue came to see me was to help them form an overview of their individual sexual needs in relation to the other needs in their lives. How important was sex for each of them? How did it make them happy? With the help of *The Game of Desire* from Peter Gerrickens, we created a life overview for each of them. David and Sue each chose ten "Needs Cards" that represented the needs they most had in their lives at this time.

David chose:
+ Not So Much Pressure
+ Movement
+ A Nice Environment To Live In
+ Peace and Quiet
+ A Healthy Body
+ Comfort
+ Humor
+ Relaxation

They both chose:
+ Love
+ Touch

While Sue chose:
- Having Fun
- Sex
- Sharing Or Expressing Feelings
- Sunlight
- A Good Relationship With Myself
- Feeling Cozy And Warm
- Intimacy And Warmth
- Adventure Or Challenge

We took a good look at the cards and talked about what they meant to both Sue and David. As we did this, David and Sue began to see how these needs are linked. For instance, reducing stress had been very important to David after his depression and this has a clear connection with his needs for movement, looking after his health and ensuring a good domestic environment for himself. He finds it very important that his house is orderly and well-equipped. Sue saw even more clearly that she loves variety in her life, spending time with other people, and that she loves to be inspired. We talked quite a bit about the Love, Touch and Sex cards. They both agreed that they are people who like to cuddle and hug.

As we talked, David spoke of his love of Sue's liveliness and Sue showed appreciation for David's steadfastness and talked of how happy she is with him as her source of security and safety. David's depression had brought some positive things with it: Sue had become much more independent and David has learned as a result of his therapy to talk more about his feelings. Their communication has improved a great deal through all this and the relationship is more enjoyable — except for their sex life.

I then asked Sue what it means for her to have gone without sex for many years. What are her reactions to this situation? How does she deal with her frustrations? We took a look at the effect that Sue's unfulfilled sexual desire has on her behavior using the second set of cards, the "Effects Cards," from *The Game of Desire*. She went through the stack in silence and set to one side the ten cards that she most recognized in her own behavior and then gave the stack back to me when she was done. I asked her to place the cards face up and next to each other in a row so that all three of us could see them. David had to laugh when he saw the card Spending Money, because he recognized the impulse purchases Sue would sometimes come home with. He was quiet again when he read the rest of the cards and took the information they conveyed onboard. I asked Sue to put the "Effects Cards" in chronological order. What happens first when she starts to notice her lack of sexual activity? What next? She laid the cards out in the following order:

- Worrying
- Blaming Others
- Bad Mood
- Suppressing Feelings

- Starting Arguments
- Eating Too Much Or Too Little
- Spending Money
- Not Using My Good Qualities.

We went through the cards one by one. Sue mentioned that she had been worrying more and more over the last years, and especially since the talk with her friends. What should she do? How could she deal with her sexual desires?

When she asked herself these questions she noticed that her thoughts immediately went to David. No matter how she looked at it, the truth was that because David could no longer satisfy her she had the tendency to blame him for the situation. She knows that is not fair as she completely understands that there is nothing he can do about it. They have tried so much already and nothing seems to work. I asked her what she feels when she is worrying. She said that she feels guilty, frustrated and angry. I then gave her the third stack from the game, the [effects on the] "Feelings Cards," and asked her to pick any cards that she recognized in her situation. Sue was surprised at the number of cards she chose:

- Tense Or Stressed
- Left In The Lurch
- Sad
- Unattractive
- Rejected
- Powerless
- Guilty
- Trapped
- Unfulfilled Or Empty

Wow" she said, "I had no idea I had so many feelings! It's no wonder that I've been buying so many new clothes lately!"

The side-effect
of unfulfilled need

It's quite common to underestimate the effect that unfulfilled needs and desires can have on us. On the surface it can seem like everything is just fine, but underneath, feelings and frustrations start to build up. These suppressed emotions can, whether we like it or not, start to have lives of their own and they can start to manifest themselves in all sorts of ways. Many compensate for important life needs being unfulfilled for long periods of time by compensating other needs. These needs are often more superficial and ultimately do not really fulfill the underlying need. Sue offers us an example as she compensates for her unfulfilled sexual needs by substituting with a need to shop. Meanwhile, the unfulfilled need doesn't go away.

I asked Sue to divide the "Feelings Cards" into two groups, one group for feelings that arise as a result of the absence of sex in her life and the other group for her feelings about David. The no-sex group contained

+ Frustration
+ Unfulfilled Or Empty
+ Unattractive
+ Rejected
+ Left In The Lurch
+ Powerless
+ Sad

As she rearranged the cards, David broke in and started to defend himself. He thought it was unfair that Sue had feelings of being left in the lurch and rejected. It isn't his fault that he doesn't feel like having sex anymore. They'd talked about this so much! He can't just decide to suddenly increase his sex drive, and poof it happens! He is going to have a loss of libido as a side-effect as long as he is on medication!

After this outburst, I asked David about his feelings surrounding not being able to have sex and the fact that Sue misses it. I gave him the "Feelings Cards" and David chose a number of cards that were the same as Sue's:

+ Frustration
+ Tense Or Stressed
+ Trapped
+ Powerless

Along with those that matched Sue's, he chose:

+ Inferior
+ Sad
+ Depressed

We then stopped and acknowledged David's feelings: he feels like he is not really a whole man since he can't give Sue the satisfaction she desires. He feels like a failure. He feels sad when he thinks about the situation, and above all, he feels trapped. He has to keep taking antidepressants for his depression and as a result he feels like there is nothing he can do about the situation.

I then asked David what he does when he and Sue argue about the lack of sex in their relationship. He told me that he has a tendency to retreat into his own world. He focuses on his work or sits for hours in front of the computer so that Sue will leave him in peace. I asked what would happen if Sue managed in some way to have her needs for sex fulfilled? What would be different between them? Sue reached down and immediately pushed the Absence of Sex feeling stack to one side and focused on her feelings for David. She said she wasn't sure, but she thought that her feelings of rejection and being left in the lurch would no longer be present. Ultimately there is no reason to blame David for something he can't do anything about and as a result she would not feel guilty anymore. Her feeling of powerlessness would disappear as well as her sadness. Sue was surprised at the magnitude of the emotional effect this change would have.

When asked, David imagined that some of his stress would disappear as well as his feelings of being trapped and powerless if Sue was sexually satisfied. If nothing else, she would stop nagging him about it and would leave the whole subject alone. David also thought that he would feel a lot less sadness. He wasn't so sure about his feelings of inferiority or frustration, or his depression. "On the other hand, I'm still a proud and honorable man and that is surely enough," he laughed.

At the end of the exercise they both said that they were surprised at the impact that Sue's unfilled desire has on her, and on their relationship. I asked them how open they were to considering possible solutions that would allow Sue to have an active and fulfilling sex life. Sue responded: "Yes, listen, I knew of course why we chose you as a coach. I'd read that you are open to unconventional forms of relationships and connections and I'd be interested to know what options there might be." David joked: "Sure, let's just find a gigolo! It's a fun idea, but if I really consider it I'd be horrified." We agreed to discuss different options in the following session.

> *Making a judgement is what happens*
> *when you discount the other*
> *ninety-nine percent of the possibilities.*
> — FROM THE DAILY THOUGHT

The path to the desired solution

> *The important thing is not to stop questioning.*
> —ALBERT EINSTEIN

It is a real art to be able to open ourselves to new ideas, especially if they appear frightening or impossible when we first hear them. Increasingly, more of us are discovering, though, that the rigid concepts we grew up with do not (any longer) work for us, or are blocking our paths. We require a certain element of courage if we want to be able to look at possibilities that may lie outside our normal frames of reference. We also require courage to look at what really is — to acknowledge that our current situations may not be entirely satisfactory, although we've tried to fix them. To create a new situation requires courage too, as well as creativity. We need to be able to creatively and freely brainstorm and to be able to set our old thought patterns and current woes to one side.

David and Sue had worked on finding a solution to their lack of sexual relations for years and had finally come to a dead end. The coaching conversations have helped them to step back and take a look at their lives and to think about what they really want. Sue does not want to go through the rest of her life without sex, but she also doesn't want to end her relationship with David. With the single exception of the fact that they don't have sex, she has nothing to complain about in her relationship. She's happy with David and loves him very much. David does not want to lose Sue for anything in the world and as for sex… well, if it's so important to her then maybe it's worth considering alternatives. He loves her, and "isn't it a sign of true love that we're willing to make sacrifices?" he asks.

The next time we met up we had a brainstorming session and came up with all sorts of possibilities to solve the situation. Nothing was too crazy to consider and we put all ideas on the table without judgement. Sue could:

+ go out to the pub and seduce someone for a one-night stand
+ hire a professional male prostitute
+ find an ongoing lover
+ seduce one of her colleagues during a business trip
+ rent sex films and buy some sex toys
+ go to a swingers club
+ seduce the parcel delivery man

As the list grew, the ideas became increasingly absurd, and the more we all laughed. When the list was long enough, we considered the pros and cons of each idea. It became rapidly apparent that Sue is not interested in simply having sex with anyone and everyone. She wants to be intimate with someone who she feels good about and with whom she can share more than just sex. David felt threatened by this idea. For him Sue visiting a male prostitute would be simplest. Then it would be clear: this is about sex and nothing else. Sue understood his thinking, but explained that she needs more than sexual contact, at the very least she needs to be friends with someone before she can have sex with them. After going back and forth for a while, they finally settled on the idea of trying to find a sexual partner for her via the Internet. Ideally it would be someone in exactly the same situation and who understands what they were doing and why. That would also lower the chances of a single man wanting more.

We stopped then and considered David and Sue's concerns. He was afraid that Sue would eventually fall in love with the other man. That is not something that would work for him. He also wants to meet the man. He wasn't prepared to just let any man touch Sue; it had to be someone he trusted. Also, he didn't want to feel left out, so he asked to be part of the search. For Sue, it was crucial that she would have full insight into the personal situation of the potential lover. She did not want to create problems in an existing relationship and only wants to be involved in a fully open and honest situation. David was prepared to try, but he asked for a veto right. If it really didn't work for him, he wants to be able to say "stop" and know that he will be heard and respected. Sue agreed to this on the condition that they would try it for six months. They agreed to put together a profile and post it to a dating site for complementary and/or polyamorous relationships.

Discovering through experience

Courage is carrying on when you've discovered
that there is a chance you can lose
—T. KRAUSE

Weighing options and talking them through is always a good idea when experimenting with a new situation. What are the advantages of a particular decision? What are our needs and what are our partners needs? What is important for each of us? How can we avoid as many difficulties as possible? One way is to use our intuition as we look after our own needs and listen to and acknowledge the concerns of others. It can be hard to achieve an ideal balance, though, as it's not really possible to know how things will play out in reality. Something that seems completely logical and straightforward can suddenly turn into an obstacle and what seems like an impasse can in reality be easily surmountable. The only way to find out is to try!

A month later I saw David and Sue again. In the interim, they had joined an online dating site and some men had responded to Sue's profile. There were a few responses that were clearly off base, but most of them were serious. There were two replies in particular that stood out. One was from an art gallery owner whose wife had undergone surgery for a serious injury, and who had subsequently lost all interest in sex. The other was from a journalist whose wife could no longer enjoy sex after a life-threatening illness left her paralyzed. Sue had decided to engage in e-mail correspondence with both of them to try to obtain a better impression. I asked how their search was going. David and Sue looked at each other and laughed. They had both found it quite exciting. Dating via the Internet was something they had read about but it was another story to do it themselves. They were both surprised at how fun it was. The atmosphere at home had also changed for the better now that they were working together to find a solution. The pressure had been released from the situation and they were having fun together again. Still, David was a bit fearful about how he would feel when it came down to Sue meeting someone. Anyway, he agreed to move to the next step.

Dating and meeting online

Many people have discovered that online dating works best when you meet the person sooner rather than later. For most of us, e-mail is not enough when it comes to deciding on a sexual contact as we need physical compatibility as well. A person's profile on a dating site can offer a glimpse of someone's personality and what is important for them; but meeting the person face-to-face can be an important part of our overall impressions. Someone can seem agreeable enough via e-mail and yet when we meet them we can be instantly turned off (or turned on!) for a wide variety of reasons. Often, we can tell in the first few minutes after meeting someone whether we are interested or not.

Sue and David decided to go together on dates with both the gallery owner and the journalist. It turned out that David found the gallery owner rather egocentric and he did not appreciate the way he made his sexual interest in Sue so blatantly obvious. Sue found him pleasant enough, but she wanted to respect David's feelings, so they made no further contact with him. The meeting with the journalist, Paul, went much better though. Sue was already impressed with his e-mails as she found the way he spoke lovingly of his wife very heartwarming. His wife, Chisa, had been wheelchair bound for years. Her paralysis started in her lower body and was slowly making its way upwards. It was now clear that she would not survive. Chisa was aware of the e-mail contact Paul had with Sue, but said she would rather not meet Sue. On the other hand, Chisa did not want to limit her husband's happiness. She had already received so much support from him and his life had been changed by her illness almost as much as hers. Chisa agreed to give Paul the space to enjoy the company of another woman, but wanted to distance herself from it. Sue immediately felt that these were two people who fostered a great amount of integrity in their relationship.

Sue found Paul very attractive, and David thought Paul to be quite a sound fellow. They had all agreed to let each other know via e-mail what their impressions were.

After their e-mail discussion, they all decided to explore things further. Sue and Paul arranged a few dates where they met for a coffee and a chat and eventually they decided to spend an evening out at a local health spa. That way they could be a bit closer to each other in a relaxed atmosphere with less clothing on. They ended up giving each other a short kiss in the shower, and later on in the car they enjoyed a more extended kiss. They both realized they wanted more. Paul rented a hotel room for the following Friday. Sue was very nervous as the evening for their date approached, but also very excited. David needed to work until 11 that night and had arranged for a baby-sitter. David and Sue had agreed that Sue would be home by 12 and that she would practice safe sex, even though Paul had a vasectomy. They also agreed that Sue would not tell David any details of their lovemaking but would only tell him whether she had enjoyed herself, felt satisfied and/or good about it.

When David arrived home from work he found Sue sitting on the couch in her bathrobe with a glass of wine in her hand, rosy cheeks and shiny eyes. He had mixed feelings about seeing his wife like this, but his curiosity and his love for her prevailed. "You had a good time," he observed. "That's great. Was he any good? No, don't tell me, I don't want to know. Let's leave it at that."

Privacy

What we tell, or don't tell, each other about our contacts with others is very individual. Some partners want to know all the details, others would rather not know anything. Some don't even want to know when their partners have had contact with someone else as they would rather not risk any potential pain. It's easier that way. Others want to know generally what is going on but let their partners keep the details for themselves. Eventually we all find what works best for us by respecting our partners wishes and sometimes by trial and error.

Sue and David had agreed that the three of them would meet up after the first sexual encounter to see how to proceed. Paul was deeply impressed with David's courage and willingness to meet him, and told him so. That was good for David to hear, and he felt seen, acknowledged and involved as a result. The three of them agreed that Sue and Paul would see each other every other week. Sue and Paul would also keep their e-mail contact to a minimum, no more than a couple of times a week. David did not want Paul to come too close, a request that Paul assured him he would honor. Paul told David that the last thing he wanted was to come between him and Sue. He respected David much too much to do that and he loved his own wife too much to contemplate such a thing.

David and Sue had little contact with me during this period. They sent me a few e-mails to keep me informed but felt no need for any further coaching until a few months later, when David requested an appointment. When they came to see me, David told me that Sue now wanted to have sex with Paul without condoms. David was not happy about this. It was against the agreement they had made. Sue thought it was nonsense to keep using them as she hated the smell of latex, Paul was sterilized and they had no sexual contact with others. There was no reason to keep using them.

I asked David if he could express what was going on for him. What was the real issue? He told me that the thought of Paul having unprotected sex with Sue horrified him. He felt like no condom between Paul and Sue would be just too intimate for him to bear. Allowing Sue to have sex with no condom would, for him, feel like he was completely giving his wife away to another man. I challenged him gently on this. "Haven't you done that already if you really look at it? Sue has a sexual relationship with someone else. She is sharing her sexuality with someone else, being orgasmic with him. So what is really going on? What's upsetting you?" I asked. David became emotional. In the conversation that followed he realized that, for him, the condom was a symbol for a process of release. He and Sue had always enjoyed sex without using condoms. By insisting that Sue and Paul use condoms, he felt that somehow his own lovemaking with Sue was special, something reserved for them. That difference would no longer be there if Paul and Sue had condom-free sex. Paul would replace him in that regard. For David, allowing Paul and Sue to have condom-free sex also meant that he was releasing any hope of ever having a normal sex life with Sue again. He would be finally acknowledging to himself that he, Sue's husband, could no longer fulfill this role for her.

This was an intense session for David. He spoke extensively about his feelings and as a result he made room inside himself to come to a place of peace. Sue was happy to give David all the time he needed to get used to the idea of her having condom-free sex with Paul. She would only do this if and when he could truly feel OK with it. As a result of this acknowledgement, David moved through his resistance much faster than expected, and ultimately gave his approval for Sue and Paul to have sex *au naturell*.

In a following session we spoke about a number of practical issues such as "What do we say to Lucy, our daughter?" Until this point, Paul and Sue had always met in a hotel but over the months this had turned into a costly exercise. As a temporary solution it had been excellent but was not sustainable in the longterm. Sue had invited Paul over to her house a few times when David was out and Lucy was playing at a friends. However the contact with Paul had changed over the months and was now more of an intimate friendship. In a certain way, Sue was starting to love Paul, although it was different from the love she felt for David. David is her life partner, her great love and the father of her child. However, Sue thought she'd like to be able to bring Paul more into her life. She was getting sick of the secrecy around Lucy. Imagine if Lucy came home early and met Paul just as he was getting ready to go home? How could they come up with a way of dealing with Lucy to avoid such an unpleasant scenario?

What do you tell the children?

Experience shows that children accept as normal what their parents accept as normal, even in the realm of intimate relationships. We pass on many of the values and norms that we have learned as a result of our upbringing, culture and society to our children. Our children are very sensitive and know exactly what is happening with us, including tension between parents. They learn by seeing rather than by simply being told. So if they see people who love each other hugging, then they learn that it's normal for people to hug each other. If they see that we love more than one person and don't make a fuss of it, then children accept multiple loving as natural too. It's mostly adults who make a big deal of alternative relationships, not children. It can be trickier though when children are older, especially as they reach their teenage years. Not all teenagers are comfortable with knowing the intimate details of their parents' love lives, especially if their parents are unconventional. Peer pressure can be enormous. Ultimately, though, children care deeply about their parents and if there is an accepting, open and normal atmosphere around parents' intimate relationships, even teenagers will often become more at ease and accepting over time.

David began to feel more relaxed about the relationship between Paul and Sue and was open to their meeting on a more regular basis. David and Sue also decided to ask Paul to come visit from time to time so that Lucy would get to know him in a natural way. Slowly, the whole family began to get used to the fact that Paul was a part of Sue's life.

In the meantime, Sue had taken over the spare room and created her own space with a comfortable chair, a bookcase and a small altar with candles as well as a sofa bed. Once in a while, she retreated into this room to meditate or to spend time with Paul; and Lucy soon learned that this was her mother's space where she was not to be disturbed. David thought that this was an excellent solution.

THE MANY FACES OF LOVE

I can understand companionship.
I can understand bought sex in the afternoon.
I cannot understand the love affair.
— GORE VIDAL

What is love? Is all love the same or are there different kinds of love? It's not only Gore Vidal who is confused! Both ancient tradition and modern research appear to confirm that there are a number of different kinds of attraction and connection that we use the word "love" to describe. For instance, the ancient Greeks had at least three different words for love:

1. EROS (ἔρως) — passionate love
2. AGAPE (αγάπη) — general affection or holding someone or something in high regard.
3. PHILIA (φιλία) — friendship and loyal love, often referred to as 'virtuous love'

Modern science seems to some extent to agree with the ancient Greeks. In 2004, the anthropologist and human behavior researcher Dr. Helen Fisher proposed that we, as a human species, have three core brain systems related to love. These are:

1. LUST — the sex drive
2. ATTRACTION — the early stage of romantic love
3. ATTACHMENT — the long-term bonding with another person

One of the most profound, and ultimately challenging, insights that can be derived from the understanding that there are different kinds of love is that we can feel different kinds of love for different people simultaneously. So we can feel sexual attraction to one person, romantic love for a second and a long-term loving connection to a third all at the same time. Science is showing us that "multiloving" is not strange or wrong, it's simply how our brains work.

The difficulty is that many people have been taught that sexual love and romantic love can only be found in monogamous relationships. In reality, this is often not the case as the statistics on infidelity so clearly demonstrate. So does this point to a fundamental moral weakness in our society? Or, is our view of love out of touch with not only our biological reality but also our cultural reality?

Traditionally in Europe, and by extension the Americas, marriage, as an institution, was not the place to have one's sexual needs fulfilled. Marriage was primarily a construction designed to ensure that families, clans and tribes could make beneficial alliances that would create strong economic ties and/or political connections. Women weren't necessarily expected to love their husbands and vice versa. As for sexual needs? They were satisfied elsewhere once the requisite children had been produced. Of course men often had far greater rights than women when it came to sexual choices.

It's only fairly recently that we've started to believe that romantic love plus sexual passion should be met by the same person. The idea that intimate love should only be expressed within the confines of a monogamous relationship has become the status quo. Yet more and more people are beginning to question the validity of this received wisdom. Open relationships challenge these relatively new traditions by accepting as normal the practice of both men and women seeking sexual variety in their lives while maintaining the strong bond of love between primary partners. In many ways, people who are practicing a polyamorous lifestyle are simply acknowledging that our ancestors knew more than we sometimes give them credit for when it comes to love. The difference is that the majority of modern open relationships are practicing polyamory in ways that allow women, as well as men, the freedom to enrich their lives by extending their expressions of love.

Questions you can ask yourself

+ How do I view the different kinds of love?
+ What agreements have I made with my partner about love and sex? How do these agreements feel to me right now?
+ How do I handle feelings of love and attraction to someone other than my partner?
+ What do I allow myself in a relationship, and why?
+ What does sexuality mean to me? To my partner?
+ What values and norms in the area of love, intimacy and sexuality was I brought up with?
+ What values and norms in the area of love, intimacy and sexuality have I passed on to my children?

Tips for a complementary sexual relationship

- Dare to think outside the box. Let your imagination and fantasies run wild. Brainstorm with your partner. Be creative.
- Include your partner(s) in what you want to do and make choices together that everyone involved can feel good about. Be open about how you feel.
- Dare to explore. You only know what something is like once you've tried it. Remember that fantasy and reality are not always the same thing.
- Take both your own and your partner(s) boundaries into consideration.
- Experiment safely.
- Enjoy and appreciate what you and your partner have between you.

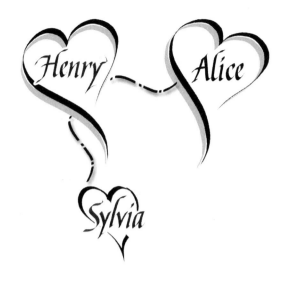

11

When Worlds Collide:
Open vs. Secret Relationships —
Henry

You are on a business trip and you meet an amazing woman. You weren't really look-ing, but you both feel attracted to each other the moment you meet. You are married, and you and your wife have agreed to an open relationship, so there's no problem there. As time goes on though, you find out that your new lover is in fact in an unhappy marriage, and that she has been meeting you in secret. So, what happens when you are in an open relationship and find yourself involved with someone who wants to have a secret affair? Does this work for you?

Henry found himself in this predicament.

Henry, forty-nine, is having a complementary relationship with Sylvia, forty-one. Henry has been happily married with Alice, forty-five, for fifteen years and they have agreed to an open relationship. They have no children. Their relationship agreement allows them both the space to express and act on their feelings for other people. Henry and Alice have each been involved in a number of relatively long-term rela-tionships with others during their marriage. They have no secrets with each other and are open and transparent about their relationships.

169

Sylvia is married to Nelson, and they have two young children. Sylvia has a challenging management position with a housing firm. Her marriage works well as far as having a family is concerned, but it doesn't provide her much more than that. Her husband is a fair enough friend, they share a house together, but their sex life is basically nonexistent. Sylvia's husband seems quite satisfied with the marriage. Sylvia, however, is quite dissatisfied with it, and yet she does not want to divorce. Her own parents had divorced when she was growing up and she is loath to make her children experience that too. So, Sylvia has decided to stick with her marriage until the children leave home. In the meantime, she satisfies herself secretly with sex and excitement elsewhere. She'd just ended such a relationship when she met Henry.

Henry and Sylvia first met at a three-day management seminar. They both felt an enormous attraction for each other from the very start. It was a residential course and on the last evening it became clear to both of them that there was a strong erotic tension between them. Henry had told Sylvia on the very first evening about his open relationship with Alice, and Sylvia eventually talked about her life with Nelson.

Sylvia talked about her dismal marital situation, and that her husband knows nothing of her affairs. Reluctantly, Henry agreed to continue their relationship, as he really enjoyed being with Sylvia; plus, her marital agreements were her business, right?

Now, the initial storm of passion between them has begun to abate and Henry's desire to see Sylvia is waning. When they are together they have a great time and Henry really enjoys Sylvia's company. However, Henry is beginning to have mixed feelings about the situation and his feelings of discomfort are increasing. On the one hand, he is very attracted to Sylvia and her eagerness to experiment and explore new sexual experiences with him. On the other hand, he is beginning to feel a sense of unpleasantness between them. He's not sure where this is coming from but he's looking less and less forward to their outings and dates. Still, whenever they meet, Henry's concerns seem to simply melt away and he fully enjoys himself. But, these feelings of doubt are beginning to really disturb him, so he makes an appointment to visit Leonie to see if she can help him find clarity.

Secrets and open relationships

The foundations for open relationships contrast with those for secretive relationships. In an open relationship the partners do not have secrets. They know about each other's complementary partners, friends with benefits or people they are in love with and they speak honestly with each other. On top of this, they make space for each other's explorations. Respect, openness, honesty and acceptance are important values here. In fact, almost always, a sustainable, open relationship can only exist if these values are at the heart of it.

A secret relationship has a very different base. The underlying beliefs tend to be that looking after self, enjoying excitement, and enjoying sexual attention from another partner are all things that can only be achieved through nondisclosure and lying.

The contradiction between the two relationship systems becomes very apparent when we decide to maintain an ongoing complementary relationship with someone who is cheating. We can find ourselves caught between honoring our own carefully thought out boundaries and colluding with the unscrupulousness of the cheating partners. Eventually this conundrum creates inner turmoil, even if it manages to avoid outer drama. Collaborating on someone else's lie can almost feel like stepping developmentally backwards, back to a time when we might not have been so sincere in our authenticity. Dishonesty robs time and energy.

During the first coaching session, we worked on helping Henry become clearer about the underpinnings of his relationship with Sylvia. He told me that the main attractions of the relationship, apart from the sex, are that he easily talks about his work with her and that they share the same sense of humor. He also enjoys the feeling that she seems to learn a lot from him, both sexually and experientially. This differs from his relationship with Alice, which is much more equal in that regard. Their journey towards an open relationship has been a joint one and many times Alice is one step ahead of him, both intellectually and emotionally.

We then looked at what is bothering Henry in his relationship with Sylvia. One of Henry's main irritations stems from Sylvia's complaints about her husband and his shortcomings. Henry sometimes has the impression that there is nothing good Sylvia can say about Nelson. Henry has confronted Sylvia with this, and has asked her why she stays with Nelson if nothing is good enough about him. Only then does Sylvia nuance herself and point out some things she likes about Nelson. Henry has made it clear to Sylvia that it doesn't make her any more attractive to him when she speaks in such a negative fashion about her husband. He also has challenged her to take responsibility for her marriage and to change the things that bother her or to do something about the things that aren't working.

Henry revealed that for Sylvia, receiving this feedback is a new experience. She's used to being very negative about her husband to her lovers. It almost seems like the darker the picture, the easier to justify cheating — to her lovers and to herself. It is strange for her to hear that Henry won't have any of it, just as it is strange for her to hear Henry speaking so lovingly and admirably about his wife. Sylvia can't really understand why Henry would spend time with her if his life was so great at home. Apparently, the only way she can make sense of this behavior is to assume that there must be something wrong with his relationship with Alice, although Henry assures her there isn't.

The influence of our values and beliefs

Many of us unintentionally assume that others think and feel the same way we do. Sometimes, we view life through the filters of our own experiences. Often, we notice this when we talk with our friends, as the advice they give is frequently based on their own values and beliefs as well as their own personal expectations and needs. They say things like "I'd leave him if I were you" or "I can't understand how you can still be with him, I certainly couldn't." Many times, our friends do try to put themselves in our shoes, but they base their reactions on their own points of view. Very often the advice they give does not really work because although their solutions may make sense to them, their ideas may not work for us.

This is exactly what is happening with Sylvia and Henry. Sylvia is cheating because her relationship at home is not working well and she is trying to energize her life through contact with other men. So it seems very strange to her that a man that she is spending time with would have a good relationship at home. Many people think, just like Sylvia, that this is impossible. The idea that someone could be completely satisfied with his or her partner, and at the same time enjoy being with others is outside their frames of reference.

Henry, however, is stuck in the same trap. He is assuming that Sylvia sees the world as he does. He is irritated by Sylvia's negativity about her husband because Henry's relationship with Alice is quite positive. In reality, he is crazy about his wife and loves their relationship and wants everyone to know about it, including Sylvia. He doesn't see that his behavior most likely makes Sylvia feel quite uncertain, uncomfortable and to some extent judged.

IMPOSED MORALITY
VERSUS INNER TRUTH

When the Tao is lost, there is goodness.
When goodness is lost, there is morality.
—LAO TZU

One of the most fundamental concepts presented in the *Tao Te Ching* (an ancient Chinese text full of great wisdom) is the understanding that imposed, external moral authority often appears when people's own sense of authenticity is either lost or suppressed. According to this text, the intention behind moral codes is, all too often, not to make us better persons, but instead to control us and make sure we act in a way that benefits those in power. The sad fact is that the very people who preach the strictest moral codes are many times those who are the most flagrant transgressors. One does not need to look too far to find glaring examples of this. Politicians and clergy are, unfortunately, frequently practicing the opposite of what they preach. Nowhere is this more obvious than in the field of relationships. Whether it's a cheating president or a Catholic bishop who has fathered a child, it's all too obvious that the powerful forces of both sex and love are often simply not compatible with what the people in power preach to the masses.

So what should we do? Simply ignore moral codes altogether? Pick and choose amongst what's offered and follow what seems right? Create our own moral guidelines? Interestingly, both the *Tao Te Ching* and many contemporary self-development paths encourage us to stop believing in the concept of morality at all. Instead of relying on external sets of rules defining what is right and what is wrong, they direct us to find ways of discovering our own inner truths. They encourage us to get in touch with our own goodness and to operate from that place of internal peace and stillness. Ironically, every organized spiritual tradition emphasizes the need to find inner stillness — whether through meditation, prayer, pilgrimage or contact with nature — and to act from that point.

A particular issue for anyone who is considering a non-monogamous lifestyle is that, by definition, they are acting in a way that most traditional Western moral codes condemn. Most people do not want to live their lives feeling like they are sinful. If someone decides to reject the prevailing moral codes there is usually a very good reason. Learning to live with the reality of conscious loving relationships to multiple partners or to one partner in ways that are authentic, congruent and coherent, and where all parties are treated with respect and dignity, can be a challenging and rewarding path of growth, awareness and personal fulfillment.

Discovering our own values and beliefs

It can be very helpful to know what our own values and beliefs are. Our inherited beliefs can greatly influence our lives; however, we can interpret these beliefs as obstructive or unhelpful when they are in conflict with our own education and experiences. When this happens it can be worth asking ourselves questions such as:

* What do *I* really think about this?
* What are *my* values and beliefs?
* How would *I* most like to deal with this situation?

In the beginning of his relationship with Alice, Henry discovered that it was quite difficult to tell his friends and his family about his open relationship. During this period, he lived an apparently "normal" life as far as the outside world was concerned. It was only after his parents passed on that he felt free enough to be honest about his choice of relationship model. Alice, on the other hand, had a much more liberal upbringing and found it easier to be candid about her private life. Over the years, she has really helped Henry to discover his own truth, and to express it.

Sylvia's reaction when she saw how well Henry's relationship with Alice worked has been a real eye-opener for Henry. He now realizes how much he has changed, and that his values and beliefs are quite different from when he was younger. When he saw Sylvia's reaction, he took the time to speak with her at length about his relationship and the values that are so important to him now. After some initial confusion, Sylvia expressed her admiration for Henry and the open relationship he's committed to; and Henry enjoyed the feeling of appreciation and acknowledgement that this realization gave him. He then noticed that Sylvia started to talk about her relationship in a different way and she started to explore ways to work on her marriage. Henry encouraged Sylvia in this process and looked forward to moving their relationship towards less secrecy and more honesty.

However things seemed to come to a standstill with Sylvia after only a couple of months. It appears that Sylvia did tell her husband about her contact with Henry, but not the details. As far as her husband knows, Henry and Sylvia met at the workshop and became friends, but he knows nothing about their sexual relationship. He hasn't asked any more, and Sylvia hasn't volunteered any further details. As far as she is concerned, that's just fine. The situation for Henry, however, is getting increasingly uncomfortable as lately Sylvia has been lying to her husband on the telephone in Henry's presence. Henry has also noticed, much to his chagrin, that he is being a bit harsh with her lately. It's almost as if she doesn't deserve to be treated in a friendly and polite fashion while she's lying to her husband.

As Henry better understood his own values and needs, as well as his behavior, he realized that his respect for Sylvia has diminished. At first, the attraction between them was so strong that it didn't seem so important to him that Sylvia was keeping her relationship with him a secret. Now that the relationship is somewhat calmer, Henry's ability to ignore his discomfort with the secrecy has decreased. The situation simply is not consistent with the values he's acquired during his own process of opening his relationship.

Yet, despite all of this, he still enjoys spending time with Sylvia. Do the benefits outweigh the disadvantages?

The balance of life wheel

It's quite normal to be unsure about a relationship or choices that will have a large impact on our lives. One way to create clarity in such a situation is to take a step back and look at our lives from a distance.

To gain some longer-term perspective — and to see the benefits that making difficult choices can have — we focus on outcomes and consequences, but also on the effects our choice(s) will have on the overall priorities in our life. So instead of wondering what can go wrong, we can ask ourselves question like:

- ✦ Am I doing things that are important for me?
- ✦ What am I spending time on?
- ✦ How do I make sure that I'm doing the things I really want to do?

A tool that can help us create an overview of these priorities is the "balance of life wheel" exercise. On a sheet of paper we draw two circles that we will divide up into sections or pie slices where each slice represents a priority. One wheel reflects our current life and one wheel reflects our ideal life.

Henry tried this exercise. After he drew his "today" circle, I asked him to compare it with his ideal world while focusing on the question "What is important for me right now?" As Henry started to sketch in the pie slices of his ideal world circle he saw that what he really wants to do is allocate more time to his psychology studies. His studies are his investment in his own future. He also wants to spend more time with his friends. He realizes that if he wants to expand both the "study" and the "friends" portions that, unless he reduces other things such as time with Alice, there really isn't a lot of room left for Sylvia. As he filled in the second pie wheel, Sylvia was the last portion to be filled in — and there was little room left for her at that point. Henry was genuinely surprised when he saw his second drawing as he suddenly understood that Sylvia was not as important to him as he thought she was. She is fun, the sex is good and she's a bit of a morale booster, but how important is she for him when compared to the other parts of his life? It was food for thought.

Questions you can ask yourself

+ What is important for me in a relationship? What behavior can I tolerate and what is unacceptable?
+ What are my own values?
+ How important are my values when it comes to a complementary relationship? Are they essential or do I simply ignore them?
+ How true to myself am I in my current relationships?
+ What would I never dare to tell my friends/families/colleagues about my relationship(s)? Why?
+ What can I learn in a complementary relationship that I can't in my current one?

Tips for complementary relationships

+ Try not to make assumptions about how someone else sees the world. Proactively compare your assumptions and expectations with the other person's to see if they align.
+ Remember that everyone is different and everyone has their own cache of experiences.
+ Be aware of your own expectations and how you react. Do you react to what is actually happening? Or, do you react to what might happen in the future?
+ Be prepared to discover. It can be helpful to view a relationship as an ongoing journey rather than a goal. Enjoy the trip and remember that things don't always go as you might have imagined — they may go better!
+ Be alert, and vulnerable. Falling into potholes and climbing out of them are all part of traversing new terrain.
+ Be thankful for what is and concentrate on enjoying the positive.

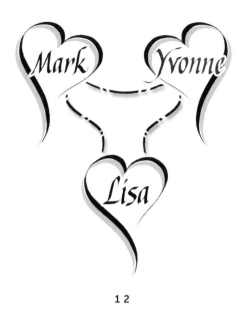

12

The Triad —
Mark, Yvonne and Lisa

You've been with your partner for decades and your children are grown and have left home. You each have your own job and social circle and are both quite independent. Emotionally, you both know you can love more than one person but you'd never really spoken to each other about this. Over the years there had been connections with other people but they never lasted. You were each aware of your partner's attractions to other people but you never really talked to each other about them. And then, something happened, and you had to talk about it. As a result, you opened up your relationship and an intense time followed where developments were fast and furious. Can your relationship of two realistically expand into a relationship of three?

Mark, Yvonne and Lisa have been working through the ups and downs of this new territory for a few years now.

Mark, fifty-one, and Yvonne, fifty-three, have known each other since they were students and have been married for twenty-six years. They have three grown children who have since moved to their own homes. Mark and Yvonne were two free spirits who met at a music festival. Neither of them had been looking for a partner at the time as they both were on journeys of growth and self-discovery. Nevertheless, they soon fell in love and moved in together. They continued to pursue their own lives when it came to their jobs, friends and social activities, and to a large extent they left each other to their own personal choices. When Yvonne became pregnant with their first child, they decided to get married. A formal wedding with traditional vows didn't seem to reflect their relationship or their lifestyles, so they opted for a more relaxed handfasting ceremony (a non-religious celebration, usually held outdoors, where guests decorate the couple's clasped hands with ribbons) instead.

Mark and Yvonne have always, each in their own way, been attracted to other people. However, their busy lives as well as the children's, took up all of their attention and a monogamous marriage was all they really knew. Also, neither of them had ever learned to truly speak openly about their inner desires to anyone, much less to each other. From time to time Mark fell in love with other women. He never did much about it other than to have the odd fantasy, and these he kept to himself. He found it all too confusing and anyway as far he was concerned it felt like love and lust were private issues. Yvonne always knew what was going on — as the signs were very obvious. When Mark was in love he was not fully present and he lived in a world of his own. His relationship with Yvonne suffered a bit during these episodes as he would become a bit absent-minded and forget things, but it was nothing that Yvonne couldn't live with.

Besides, Yvonne often felt sexually attracted to other men. She fantasized and she enjoyed flirting and feeling the sexual chemistry — which gave her a real boost that she used in her daily life with the family. Mark and Yvonne carried on like this for many years and were basically satisfied with life as it was.

One day, Yvonne took things a bit further when one of her flirtations turned into more. Mark was only the third man she had ever had sex with and after so many years with him she felt like she was ready for something new — although she didn't dare admit that to Mark. Her new lover brought a whole new level of sexual challenge and discovery into her life and her secret trysts filled her with thrills and excitement; still, mutual sexual attraction was really all there was between them. Nevertheless, when Mark found out about what was going on he was furious. He was shocked when he discovered that Yvonne had been having sex with another man for eighteen months. He hadn't noticed a thing! Yvonne had been more interested in sex lately and he'd enjoyed that, but he hadn't really thought any further about why that could be. When he found out what was going on between Yvonne and her lover, it all finally made sense to him. Mark could see that Yvonne's explorations had actually benefited their own relationship. Still, his feelings of jealousy, and above all the fact that he had been deceived, overrode any positive feelings he might have allowed regarding what had occurred. So, four years ago they found Leonie and set up counseling in an attempt to save their marriage.

Some like love, some like sex

During their sessions, Mark and Yvonne had, above all, learned how to communicate with each other. In addition, Mark discovered that his jealousy was primarily based on the fear that the other man would be a better lover for Yvonne. He was also afraid that Yvonne would leave him for the other man. When he brought this out into the open, Yvonne made it clear that she loved him dearly as a lover and as a husband and that she had no intention of leaving him at all. Once he understood this, Mark's jealousy became much more manageable. Mark and Yvonne also learned how to speak to each other about their sexual desires and they discovered as a result that they had quite different feelings and views of sexuality.

For Mark, sexuality is deeply connected to intimacy and a feeling of soul connection. He can't imagine having sex with a woman that he is not in love with and for him physical intimacy can only happen when there is spiritual and emotional intimacy as well. He has a strong sense of loyalty to his wife and family and finds himself struggling whenever his heart is touched by another woman. He judges himself harshly when this happens and feels misunderstood by others who, noticing the sparks between Mark and another woman, simply jump to the conclusion that he is only after sex.

Yvonne is different. She loves sex and enjoys it for what it is, a playful and sensuous encounter between two consenting adults. If there is a strong physical attraction coupled with mutual respect, her sexual energy can flow. She enjoys a certain level of intimacy as well but this is not a prerequisite for her. On the other hand, Yvonne does feel very guilty about her desire to have sex with a man other than her husband as her Catholic upbringing makes it clear that this is shameful behavior. Her childhood catechism has indeed provoked an internal struggle as she questions whether she is a "normal" woman.

And so it was that both Mark and Yvonne found themselves confronted with the reality that their professed monogamous relationship was no longer accurately reflecting who they were. Their marriage form was beginning to create great stress for each of them and by extension, their relationship.

Relationship agreements

It's only when you display the courage to walk your own path
That your path will reveal itself to you
—PAULO COELHO

Many of us, whether we are conscious of it or not, do not really feel suited to a monogamous relationship. This is not surprising as clearly not all of us *are* monogamous. However being non-monogamous is not something most people find easy to acknowledge and feel good about. Most of us have grown up in a society that still gives lip service to the idea that monogamy is the single option for marriage and partnerships, and that marriage is the only way to form long-term relationships. So, when non-monogamous people decide to form long-term relationships they still often choose to get married, as it is the only relationship form that is legally and socially accepted. Marriage includes a presumption that we will only have intimate loving and/or sexual relationships with one partner. This is a real problem for a marriage between one or more non-monogamous partners as feelings for other people are bound to surface eventually and the assumed agreements of "one partner only" may be broken.

When this happens, we often do not know how to — and are afraid to — speak with our partners about our feelings for other people, especially when sex is involved. There are many reasons for this but two of the most common are:

1. Most of us, despite the sexual revolution of the sixties, find it difficult to speak openly and freely about our sexuality.
2. If we want to allow space for feelings and connections to others in our marriage, we may need to renegotiate our marriage agreements. This is not something that most of us know how to do, would even expect to do, or would be brave enough to do as the outcome is not certain.

However, the trends in society are unmistakable. Once we might have assumed that we would work for the same employer all our lives, whereas we now accept that job changes and further education are normal, and indeed desirable, features of 21st-century work life. Relationships are not immune to this change and the number of divorces and remarriages attest to the desire for variety and growth. But does a relationship need to end simply because of change? Or, is it possible to allow a relationship to redefine itself as each partner's needs and desires shape and reshape over time?

Before Mark and Yvonne married, they spoke with each other about what they each felt was important in a relationship. They decided to promise each other on their wedding day that they would give each other the freedom to continue to develop personally and that they would support each other in this. They would agree to be friends and they would not be each other's possession. They would maintain their individuality and did not wish to melt into each other and become a single unit. They would appreciate and support each other's uniqueness.

This relationship agreement worked for them and, indeed, over the years they both developed in different, quite separate ways. Yvonne held a number of jobs and had finally started her own Reiki and massage practice. Mark worked for various multinationals before setting up his own IT consultancy. They were both happy with how their own lives were developing and with the family they had created together. They both felt they were achieving what they had promised years ago when they got married.

During the coaching sessions, Mark and Yvonne realized that the time had come to renegotiate and renew their relationship agreement. They were both clear that they had feelings, albeit different kinds, for others and that they had not spoken of this when they created their original relationship agreement. They wanted to find ways to allow connections with others to take place while at the same time ensuring that their own relationship would not be damaged.

To start, we looked at the consequences of Yvonne's illicit trysts with her lover. Yvonne decided to stop seeing him because she and Mark both wanted to rebuild the trust between them. From that point forward, they promised each other that they would be open and honest about their feelings for others.

I then asked them to each choose ten "Behavior Cards" from *The Relationship Game*, which corresponded with their relationship goals for the coming period. They both chose Be Open And Honest With Each Other. Accept Each Other As You Are was also chosen by both, and they discovered that they each felt this meant that they would accept each other's differences and not attempt to change each other. Besides these two cards, they chose Dare To Be Vulnerable and Share Feelings And Personal Issues as aspects they would like to see in their relationship. They agreed that these skills would be necessary to be able to speak freely about intimacy and sexuality.

Their personal challenges were highlighted by Mark's choice of Release Negative Relationship Experiences and Yvonne's Work On One's Own Personal Development cards. For Yvonne, this meant a practical commitment to looking at how she could work on overcoming the influences of her strictly religious upbringing, and that she might attend some sort of course or training with other women dealing with the same issues. Mark agreed to identify and commit to a personal development practice that would allow him to become more fully present and to learn how to release old pain and energetic obstructions. They also agreed to spend at least two evenings per month together consciously communicating about and strengthening their relationship. They ended their sessions feeling significantly happier and with a sense of renewed commitment to their relationship.

Living our authenticity

Mark and Yvonne renegotiated their relationship agreement and decided to give each other the space to explore what they each really wanted in the realm of relationship and sexuality. They were fully aware as they did this that it would take time to change some of the patterns they had locked themselves into over the years. As they got started, they discovered how difficult it is to unravel patterns that are based on our childhoods. Indeed, most people experience this when they attempt to deal with deep-seated relationship behaviors. The process is not made any easier by societal pressures. We can find it quite challenging to find our inner truths, our cores. It's not only learned behavior that we need to grapple with but also countless beliefs, convictions, negative thoughts and fixed values. On top of that, our egos can definitely put up a good fight!

Do we dare allow ourselves to acknowledge what we really want? Do we dare let our partners, our families and our friends know? Do we even allow ourselves to stop and look at our desires at all? Do we dare claim our authenticity? Ultimately, we need to learn how to listen to our hearts if there is to be any hope of living a life based on who we are rather than one based on who others expect us to be. A crucial part of this task is to learn not to judge but instead to respect ourselves with all the emotions and desires that being human entails.

Being non-monogamous in an open, honest and ethical fashion is not something that, generally, our society supports or understands. That's why it is so nice to find people who can understand and support us if we choose to explore this openhearted path. However it's not always so easy to find such people in our own circle of friends and social contacts, so many people interested in polyamory use Internet forums as support vehicles. As our self-acceptance grows, however, we often find that the resistance we have experienced from our friends begins to fade away. When we radiate happiness and satisfaction with our lives and the choices we have made, others usually find it easier to accept us, even if they don't totally understand or agree with our choices.

Four years went by before Mark and Yvonne contacted me for another appointment. A lot had happened with them during those years, and they took some time to fill me in. The first year after they had renewed their relationship contract had been one of many conversations and several discoveries. They had taken the time to speak openly and honestly about all love and attractions they had secreted over the years. A great deal of clarity had been created as a result. They grew closer and could now talk with each other easily. During the second year it became clear that the time had come for a new step in their relationship. Yvonne had decided that she was ready to explore and develop her sexuality and wanted to free herself from the shackles of her upbringing. She decided to join a course specifically for women grappling with these issues. The course included the opportunity for the participants to engage sexually with trained men; and Mark encouraged her to join. As Yvonne progressed through the course she realized that she also wanted the freedom to be able to have sexual connections with men outside the course if she met someone she felt good about. After much discussion, Mark decided that he was willing to support her in her sexual explorations, even though he knew that it would not always be easy for him. This was an exciting step for Yvonne but she was cautious not to jump into it too quickly as she did not want to endanger her relationship with Mark. As she continued step by step both Mark and Yvonne found that their own sexual relationship benefited as Yvonne allowed herself to more fully embrace her sexuality. Now that they could speak openly, Mark no longer felt deceived or lied to and their mutual trust was rebuilt.

Mark was hesitant when it came to accepting another woman into his life, as he knew that his needs were different from Yvonne's — he needed intimacy and a spiritual connection as well as physical one. And then he met Lisa. The energy between them was so strong that all of Mark's reservations were blown away. He fell completely head-over-heels in love with her and both his life and Yvonne's life have been spinning as a result.

Lisa and Mark met at a workshop they attended together; and Mark was smitten from the moment they met. During the lunch break he was in a bit of a fluster and he took Yvonne to one side and mentioned that he would be interested in seeing more of Lisa. Yvonne was slightly amused at the effect Lisa clearly had on Mark and immediately understood that this was no ordinary meeting. Lisa, forty-two, is bisexual; and Mark appreciated the fact that Lisa is a self-aware and independent woman and very at ease with herself. Lisa was attracted to both Mark and Yvonne right away too, and was not shy about showing it. Yvonne encouraged Mark to invite Lisa over to their house for dinner the following weekend, as Yvonne was curious to get to know Lisa a bit better and wondered where this might be leading.

A week later it was time for their meal together. In the meantime Mark and Lisa had been e-mailing each other, and the more they got to know each other, the stronger their connection became. Mark kept Yvonne fully in the loop. When Lisa finally came in the door they all had a feeling that they'd known each other for years. They had a great evening together and they were all pleasantly surprised at the sparks that were flying between the three of them. Yvonne didn't feel like she was in love with Lisa but she did feel very comfortable with her. Yvonne's ease with her own sexuality had developed over the last few years and she stretched her experiential boundaries significantly as a result. Although she never felt sexually attracted to another woman before, she now realized that she didn't mind in the least being physically close to Lisa. Yvonne liked the idea of being with Mark and another woman at the same time, and wondered if this was the chance for one of her dreams to come true with someone that they might even see on an ongoing basis.

Over the next week Mark and Lisa spent hours on Skype and Mark and Yvonne spent hours conversing. Yvonne was happy that Mark was in love, and felt relatively unthreatened because she was included. Eventually, the three of them spent a weekend together, and had such a great time that they decided to spend every weekend together from then on. As far as they were concerned they were clearly, and officially involved in a happy three-way relationship.

Mark and Yvonne were clear that starting a relationship with Lisa would have a significant impact on their own relationship. All three of them agreed that it was important that sufficient attention be paid to Yvonne as the energy was so strong between Mark and Lisa. By spending weekends together they could make sure of this. All three of them were committed to making it work for each one of them and the first few months were a dream come true. And yet, after the fourth month had passed, all was not well. They were deeply confused, which is what brought them back to see me.

The problem, it seems, is that Yvonne recently indicated that she would like to spend a weekend alone with Mark from time to time. Mark wants none of it. He feels that they have time together during the week and that they have committed to being with Lisa at the weekends. Didn't Yvonne consciously choose to be in the triad? Would this be fair to Lisa?

Now, all of a sudden, Mark feels caught between a rock and a hard place. He does not want to hurt or upset Yvonne but neither does he want to shortchange Lisa. Mark knows that Lisa really enjoys their weekends together. She feels like she is living her dream scenario where she has relationships with a man and a woman that she loves dearly. She hates to go home every Sunday evening but has no choice as her work and house are a long way away. So what now? How can they deal with the different needs and desires between the three of the them?

The joys and challenges of a triad

A complete triad relationship, i.e. one where all three people love and have a relationship with each other, can be very fulfilling. A triad solves one of the most intractable problems faced by couples: duality. In monogamous relationships, two people deeply connect and share the level of intimacy a committed relationship can provide. Eventually, this can lead to right/wrong, will/won't, have/haven't types of interactions. Even with the best intentions, it can be quite difficult to avoid falling into these patterns, and they can often lead to rigidity and even communication breakdowns as we defend fixed positions. The triad offers us a completely different dynamic. For instance, during a difficult one-on-one interaction, a third partner can sometimes act as a loving observer. The presence of this witness can make it easier for the interacting partners to be conscious of their actions and reactions. This self-consciousness can result in more flexible, open and responsive interactions. The abundance we can experience when we are no longer looking to just one person for our intimacy can also help us to relax and allow ourselves to simply be loved. We can feel more acknowledged and affirmed and our own life energy can flow more freely and benefit everyone in our lives.

Interestingly enough, many of us discover that when we are in triads we feel more independent and free than when we are couples. This happens both on a practical and a more subtle level. Practically, it means that if one person wants to spend some time alone or with friends, they can relax knowing that the other two partners have some time to spend together. On a deeper emotional level, the partners can also discover that a triad often seeks its own energetic balance. The positive manifestation of this can be seen for example when one partner for some reason takes on a stronger, slightly dominant role. Whereas in a couple this can often degenerate into an unhealthy dynamic, a triad often rebalances itself when the other two partners support each other and counterbalance the dominating behavior. This way, each partner can support the others in turn to stay in their power; and this can help each one maintain their individuality. Often, those involved in triad relationships discover that they are far more in balance, both intellectually and emotionally, than many couples. To paraphrase a well known truism: a three-legged stool is much more stable than a two-legged one.

There is a potential downside to the triad, however, which is immediately apparent: it is a more complex arrangement. Each partner has a different set of attractions to the other two. Learning to create ways to have clarity and harmony amongst three people is definitely more work than with two people.

I asked Mark and Yvonne what the pros and cons of their triad are. Mark said it was wonderful that Lisa is such a good discussion partner with whom he can have deep conversations. They talk for hours sometimes, and Lisa often challenges him to see life from another point of view. Yvonne is delighted to see Mark so happy. She notices that he has a lot more energy and that has resulted in more positive interactions all around. She loves experimenting in bed with both of them. Yvonne also likes to go shopping with Lisa and thinks it's fun to be able to playfully team up with Lisa and tease Mark. The two women have created a special connection with each other and that feels good.

Still, they both agree that at the end of the day Mark is the glue that holds the triad together. Although Yvonne thinks Lisa is fantastic, she doesn't have the same feelings for her as she has for Mark. Yvonne is wondering if, given this imbalance, the relationship has a long-term future. She's also noticed that the intensity of the relationship can, at times, be a bit much for her. I asked Yvonne what exactly she was referring to, the relationship between her and Lisa or the relationship between the three of them? Yvonne thought about this for a second. "That's a good question," she answered. "Sometimes I'm not really sure anymore what my life looks like. On the one hand I still feel like Mark and I are a couple and that we have simply opened up our relationship to include Lisa. We've known each other for so long and we know each other so well that it's simply not possible to pretend that ours is a new relationship. On the other hand, sometimes I think that this *is* a new relationship and that the old days of just the two of us are all over. The new triad relationship is fun, but sometimes I miss just spending time with Mark and would like to spend a weekend with just him and maybe one or two of the children. It can be a bit much with all the talking, communicating and being aware of each other that happens when the three of us are together."

I then asked Mark how he views the triad and which relationship is currently getting most of his attention. He responded that the triad is his main focus. Life with Yvonne is good at the moment, but above all he looks forward to the weekends when they are all together. As far as he is concerned, spending time together with all three of them is the way to make the triad work.

185

The different relationships in a triad

There are actually four relationships in a triad, in this case between Mark and Yvonne, Mark and Lisa, Yvonne and Lisa and the three of them together. In other words, each person has three different relationships to maintain; and each has its own qualities and dynamics.

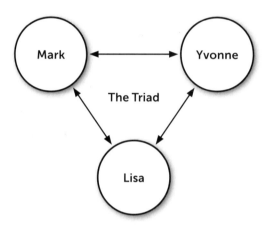

A common difficulty that many triads come across is a completely understandable desire for there to be equality amongst these relationships. This is not easy to achieve and, realistically, it is simply not possible all the time. Many things happen when a third person enters into a relationship with a couple who've been together for many years. The preexisting relationship is, in many ways, not equal to the three new ones. The original couple shares a common past including children they may have, shared projects and possessions, and their emotional connections. This history is not something that we can simply pretend does not exist. Each of the four relationships will have its own dynamic and will be different from the other ones. To add to this complexity is the fact that the emotional strength of each of the relationships is bound to be different, and will vary in intensity as time passes. Each relationship has its own special kind of love as it is a unique connection.

So, how can we reconcile these inequalities of circumstances and connections with the desire to create a fair, equitable and sustainable triad? One way is to step back and observe the situation as a creative process. In other words, instead of saying "We are a triad, how do we make it work?" we can say instead "We are in the process of creating a workable triad." This is especially useful when the starting point is an existing couple. Just because two married people have decided to open up their relationship to a new partner does not mean that the original relationship between them no longer exists. Just the opposite — often the original relationship and its qualities are the very thing that attracts the new partner in the first place. So discarding or trying to undo it for the sake of the new triad would be totally counterproductive. It can be useful to start a process where we become aware of the patterns and assumptions that have become self-evident in the original relationship, and then reexamine, adjust or shed as necessary. As we do this we can take into account the new partner and do our best to make decisions based on his or her point of view as well.

The new partner will need to accept that, indeed, he or she is joining an existing relationship. There's really no way around this and at times the new partner will feel left out. At such times it can be helpful if there is room to acknowledge and express these feelings. Sometimes all we need to do is make sure that we consciously include the new partner in whatever is happening. It's a skill that can be worth developing and it involves simply being aware of what is going on in the moment, and then providing that extra little bit of affirmation and acknowledgment that can make all the difference.

I asked Yvonne and Mark to spend a bit of time during the following week thinking about the different relationships in their triad and to find ways to describe them. I also asked them to consider what their wishes and desires are for each one of the relationships. I suggested that they share with Lisa the details of our conversation, and that they might think about inviting Lisa to join the next coaching session. Yvonne and Mark agreed.

A week later a delighted Lisa called me and said she'd like to come and have a separate coaching session with me first. Lisa talked about the highlights of her life until then and how she experienced her relationship with Yvonne and Mark. It turned out that Lisa had experienced a few problematic relationships with men that had difficulties with her bisexuality. When she turned thirty, she'd decided that she was going to be in charge of her life and was no longer going let others determine who she was. She intended to fully embrace her bisexuality and to enjoy it. During the last few years she'd had a number of concurrent relationships, both with men and women. She's enjoyed the sex but ultimately the short-term connections were not fulfilling. What she's really been longing for is deep intimacy.

When she met Mark and Yvonne for the first time she was immediately taken with Mark's openness and honesty as he spoke of his relationship with Yvonne. She was attracted to both of them although she did find it easier to interact with Mark at first. She was initially concerned about the mutual attraction between her and Mark because she didn't want to come between Mark and Yvonne. This concern was allayed when she received the invitation from both of them to come over for a meal. She screwed up her courage while talking to Mark and Yvonne and, for the first time in her life, told them her dream to be in a three-way relationship. She was overjoyed at their positive response.

Soon, Lisa's friends noticed that she was happy and full of energy and began to ask her what was going on. Was she in love? She'd already decided that she wanted to be open and honest about her relationship with Mark and Yvonne and, much to her surprise, her candidness had been met with generally positive responses as well as the inevitable "how do you arrange things in bed?" Even her parents told her that they were prepared to put their initial concerns to one side now that they saw how happy she was. They didn't totally understand what she was up to, but their daughter's happiness was the most important thing for them. This touched Lisa deeply.

When she spoke about the things that Yvonne and Mark had told her from the last session with me, she said that she had been somewhat surprised at the idea that she now had three different relationships: one with Mark, one with Yvonne and one with the two of them. As far as she was concerned she was busy with the triad — meaning the relationship with the three of them together. Now that she thinks about it, her feelings for Mark are indeed different from her feelings for Yvonne. She feels a closer spiritual connection to Mark than to Yvonne. Her attraction and connection to Yvonne is more physical and social. Lisa enjoys Yvonne's gentle and powerful femininity and sexuality. She admires Yvonne for her ability to listen without judging and the way she comes out with trenchant and pithy statements or observations that gives Lisa food for thought. Lisa's feelings for Mark are different. Mark challenges her; and the erotic charge between them is very strong. Ideally she would like to spend some time alone with Mark to explore their sexual relationship. She only dared to suggest this once, though, as she is afraid of coming between Mark and Yvonne. The last thing she wants to do is to throw a spanner into the works of their relationship. The truth is that she feels Mark and Yvonne have more rights with each other as their relationship predates hers. On top of this, they'd all agreed to spend their weekends together and she did not want to break that agreement. She fully understands that it is very important to make and keep agreements when in a polyamorous relationship. At the same time, she's begun to realize that she isn't being totally upfront with her own wishes and desires.

In the following session, Mark, Yvonne and Lisa each used a modified "Connection Wheel/Triad" drawing to view their three different relationships.

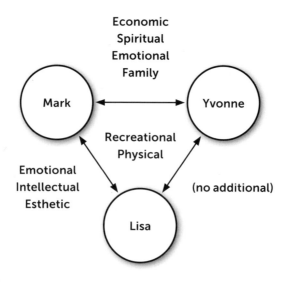

It was immediately striking to all three of them that the relationship between Yvonne and Lisa is only based on the connections that are there for the triad as a whole i.e. recreational and physical. When questioned, Yvonne shared that she does have some sense of emotional connection to Lisa. When she looked at this closer, she admitted that she doesn't feel a huge amount of trust when it comes to their relationship. She worries a bit as sometimes her interactions with Lisa can be rather emotionally loaded and draining. Sometimes she thinks Mark and Lisa should just go play and leave her in peace. But when she thinks this way, she feels mistrust for Lisa, and she feels stuck. "Mark is such a fantastic man," she told me, "and I don't want to lose him." Deep inside, she hears her own voice asking Lisa, "You're not going to take him from me, are you?" She started to cry as she admitted that she is indeed uncertain of what is going on between Mark and Lisa.

All three of them decided then that it was worth taking a closer look at what is going on with Yvonne's mistrust. When she stopped to think about it, she realized that she is confused. On the one hand she is feeling unsure about what effect Mark and Lisa's relationship will have on the relationship between Mark and herself. On the other hand she admits that in some way it would be a relief if she could simply let go and let Mark and Lisa develop their own relationship without her having to be consistently present. In fact, she would enjoy more time for herself. "Actually, I think I've forgotten the relationship with myself in all of this" she added.

Mark and Lisa had been listening carefully while Yvonne was talking. They were genuinely surprised at what they heard. A few weeks back, Lisa had sent Mark an e-mail telling him how wonderful it would be if they could spend some time together, just the two of them. Mark had simply told her that this was not in the cards. His response had been so firm that Lisa felt guilty for even having suggested the idea. After all, they had consciously started their relationship with the three of them together and here she was wanting something different. She accepted Mark's answer while assuming that Mark and Yvonne have significantly more life experience than she does, and also more skill in handling an open relationship. Yet, her intuition told her that something wasn't quite right. She felt like the situation was not totally fair and equal as Mark and Yvonne got to see each other all week long while she only got to see them at the weekends. To add to this she realized that even if they all lived together she would never be able to catch up on all the years that Mark and Yvonne spent together. How could she ever truly be equal? Sometimes, when she sees how close Mark and Yvonne are, and how much they share with each other, she gets frustrated and feels a bit left out. When she looked closely she realized that she sometimes reacts negatively and somewhat harshly to Yvonne as a result. As she spoke of this, she understood that it was not really fair of her to do this and she apologized to Yvonne, who readily accepted and gave her a hug.

Mark was surprised but relieved when he heard all this. He'd felt totally responsible for everyone over the last few months and it had started to get to him. After all, he is the one who fell in love with Lisa. He was the one who made the first advances.

Truth be told, he finally feels like he is part of the action after years of being sidelined while Yvonne enjoyed all sorts of adventures.

Mark admits that he is also afraid of the strong emotions he is feeling with Lisa even though he understands that he is suffering from a severe case of NRE. He guesses that he would be better able to keep his emotions under control if he only sees Lisa as part of their threesome time; however, this is a sacrifice. That's why he had responded so harshly when Yvonne had suggested that *she* and Mark should spend a weekend alone. The idea that Lisa would not be there upset him terribly.

Yvonne, Lisa and Mark were delighted with this session together. I suggested that when they were home they might look at how they would ideally like to spend time with each other if they weren't so afraid of what might happen. Who would spend time with whom and when? What kind of agreements would they ideally want to have?

As a result, they all agreed that it would be a good idea if twice a month, Mark and Lisa would spend a Friday evening and the following Saturday together at Lisa's flat. This way Yvonne would have some time for herself. On those Saturday evenings Mark and Lisa would then drive to Mark and Yvonne's house and they would all spend the rest of the weekend together. They would also try to ensure that Lisa and Yvonne could socialize at least once a month without Mark; and when any of Mark and Yvonne's children want to visit, Lisa would not come see them so that Mark and Yvonne could enjoy some family time together.

Three months later they came to see me again. In principle they were very happy with how things were going between them. Things seemed much more relaxed and Yvonne said she had room to breathe again. This arrangement makes it a lot easier for her to deal with Mark being madly in love with Lisa.

Mark is very happy that he can spend time alone with Lisa. In the meantime though he is beginning to see that there is another side to the coin. Lisa doesn't hesitate to confront him with his behavior, especially when they are just the two of them. The passion between Mark and Lisa is much higher than between Mark and Yvonne, but so is the amount of arguing. Mark has found himself quite frustrated at times with Lisa. When he is with Lisa he wants to enjoy their time together. He doesn't want to waste time on arguing and unpleasant discussions. Sometimes he wonders why Lisa can't be more like Yvonne and just let things be if they can't agree. Yvonne simply returns to an issue later when they've both calmed down instead of arguing it to death. He knows that Lisa is different but he's having trouble dealing with her hot reactions.

Relationship patterns and interactions in a triad

We all develop both positive and negative patterns of behavior in our relationship(s) over time. This happens naturally as we get to know each other and as we adapt our usual way of doing things to create smoother, more harmonious interactions between ourselves and our partner(s). Positive behavior patterns support us in creating energized, alive and joyful interactions. On the other hand, negative patterns can, if we are not careful, lead us into dysfunctional and energy-sapping situations. One of the unique and challenging characteristics of a triad is that the existence of these patterns is frequently highlighted as the patterns developed with one person often do not work well with another. Energy loss can also occur when we switch our attention between partners and then need to adapt to their respective, often different, ways of interacting. The key to avoiding the confusion and frustration this can create is to remain flexible, tolerant and in the here and now. The pattern-revealing dynamic in a triad can help us to become more present and open to the reality that "change is the only constant." When we base our relationships on the underlying intentions of each partner rather than how we interpret each partner's actions, we simplify and energize our relationship(s).

Each triad has unique communication and intimacy structures. Some are based on a relatively equal level of connection between the three partners while others are primarily based on one person's connection to two other people. No matter what the form, however, each one of the three people all have some kind of relationship to the other two. In practice, most successful triads have discovered that it's important that each person communicates directly with each other partner rather than via the third. In addition, it works best when all three people ensure that they are autonomous, self-aware and willing to take full responsibility for their own actions. The benefits of a triad are numerous, but to make one really work over the long-term requires a willingness to work consciously on creating healthy and conscious relationship(s).

I then turned to Lisa. She told me that she is delighted with the new agreements they have made. She thinks it is great to spend time alone with Mark once in a while. She admits that she enjoys not only discussing things with Mark but also provoking him out of his shell. She does find it difficult when he gets irritated and annoyed with her though, and often feels she's pushed him too far. Still, she never worries about their sometimes fiery discussions. She is used to standing up for herself and making things clear to others. She is a bit of a fighter, she said. It is just that sometimes Mark doesn't seem to take her seriously, and that annoys her.

Lisa has also discovered that the time she has for herself when Mark and Yvonne's children are visiting is quite nice, as it allows her time to think. The difficult discussions with Mark have made her realize that they not only have an age and experience difference, but the relationship could end if they don't find a better way to communicate. Lisa knows that the interactions can be more productive, because she and Mark communicate in a completely different way when Yvonne is present. Yvonne's softer way of being, her relaxed manner and inherent respect for others has a healing effect on both of them. Somehow, their sharp edges are softened when Yvonne is around, and they laugh more. The triad relationship is built on having fun and being relaxed with each other and Lisa realizes that she really loves it and would miss it horribly if it ended.

The atmosphere changed suddenly when Lisa said all this. Mark noticed then that although Lisa is the youngest of the three of them she is the most courageous. He too had been wondering if the whole relationship was at risk. He really doesn't want to think about this though and he is determined to make the triad a success.

I asked all three of them to take a few minutes in silence to think about their worst fears, and to write these down. I then asked them to take the fears and put them to one side. Next, without breaking their silence, I suggested that they try to get in touch with their senses of love and calmness… and finally to write down what they have the greatest sense of trust in.

Yvonne had written down that her greatest fear is that she and Mark would grow apart as a result of not having anything to offer each other any more. She then said that she most trusted that she and Mark had been together for so many years, and had already come through so much together, and that they had always managed to work things out in the end. She has a strong sense that, no matter what, they'll always find a way to enjoy life as they grow as partners. She also feels a strong soul connection between them and trusts she will always be connected to him.

Mark's greatest fear is that he won't be able to manage two relationships with two different women at the same time. He is struggling with the interaction between Yvonne and Lisa and in his relationship with each of them and it is taking more out of him than he wants to admit. His greatest trust is based on the fact that the older he gets the more he realizes that he is indeed human and fallible. His willingness to have these two relationships has allowed him to become more tolerant and more accepting of himself and his imperfections. He trusts that as long he is willing to stay open and vulnerable that he will be able to navigate his way through the challenges these relationships present.

Lisa wrote that her greatest fear is that the relationship would end. She is totally hooked on both Yvonne and Mark and she is incredibly happy to have both a man and a woman in her life. She's very afraid that the situation will implode if things start to go wrong. Her greatest trust is in her own relationship with herself. She knows that she is a strong and autonomous woman and that she enjoys challenges, and here she is in the middle of one. She's chosen to be in this situation out of her own free will. She knows that no matter what happens she will always be stronger and wiser for it.

Everyone present was touched by the wisdom and depth of their answers. The tension in the room was replaced with peace. They each decided to continue looking at how they could best help each other process these fears. A few weeks later, Mark called and told me the last session provoked a wonderful conversation between the three of them. They'd gone back and looked at what each of them had written down and talked about how they could help each other satisfy what their fears highlighted. The most important thing, he said, was that they had acknowledged the importance of each individual relationship and had also accepted that ultimately each relationship needs to stand on its own merits. If, for some reason, one of the relationships does not work out, they each agreed to work towards a gentle resolution that would not endanger the other relationships. This gave them all an enormous sense of freedom and relief and reduced the pressure on the triad. They agreed that each of them would contribute to the triad what felt right for them as individuals; and that the underlying commitment for all three of them was to grow — both personally and collectively. They also acknowledged that by freeing time for each one of them, including Mark, to spend time alone they are all better able make choices based on their own internal sense of what is best.

Mark laughed when he told me that at the end of the conversation Yvonne jumped up and said, "Enough talking already! Let's just enjoy ourselves and what we have together!"

Courage is not the absence of fear,
it is instead being able to feel fear and still follow your heart.
—DAVID DEWULF

THREESOMES AND TRIADS:
OLD AND NEW

Simone de Beauvoir, Anaïs Nin, Pablo Picasso, Salvador Dali: all are well known historical figures and all, in one form or another, were involved in unconventional relationships involving three people. No matter what the term — *ménages à trois*, threesome or triad — the combination of three people in an emotional and/or sexual relationship is a part of human history. In fact, the carvings and drawings on ancient temples from the Indian subcontinent and the Far East leave no doubt that the practice of sexual rituals amongst three people was practiced there in ancient times. What is the attraction of such an arrangement? If maintaining and nurturing a relationship with two people is work enough, why would one increase the complexity by an order of magnitude? Surely there must be significant benefits to "the constellation of three" to outweigh the inevitable difficulties of such an unconventional and complex relationship. What, exactly, are these benefits?

Many people, when questioned who benefits from a triad, would answer "the man of course!" This response is often based on two common assumptions: the first that the triad is composed of one man and two women; and the second that the fundamental purpose of the arrangement is to provide more sexual opportunities for the man in question. However, if one looks more closely at actual long-term relationships of three (as opposed to short-term sexual liaisons) the picture that emerges is rather different. Probably one of the most common triad configurations involves at least one, if not two, people who are to some degree bisexual. This makes sense since if someone is bisexual then a triad is a relationship form that provides a situation where both sides of their sexual nature can find expression.

So are there benefits to the general emotional and physical health of those in a triad compared to the partners in a couple? Many people in triads would answer with a resounding "Yes." To understand why, it can be interesting to first consider an ancient Taoist text paraphrased as, "The best sexual configuration is one between two women and a man." This text also considers the opposite scenario, i.e. two men and one woman but recommends against it as "two Yins can cooperate but two Yangs will compete." One interpretation of this portion of the text is that this energy dynamic has more to do with the personal male/female qualities of the people involved rather than their specific gender. The text further offers that each person can learn to take full responsibility for their sexual energy while at the same time enjoying a significantly increased availability of excitement and energy flow. Indeed, the anecdotal evidence tells us that the level of energy that can be created when three people engage sexually with each other is many times higher than that in a duo. When this energy is used consciously, as in the Taoist and Tantric traditions, it can be a powerful source of fuel for personal and spiritual development.

The emotional dynamics of a triad are in many ways predicated by the arrangement that the three people have created. The traditional polygamous arrangement had the man at the centre i.e. a husband and two wives where the women were subservient to the man. This scenario is something that, not surprisingly, many people today are not comfortable with as it reinforces patriarchal oppression. However, the modern version of this arrangement — a triad — is something very different. In such a threesome, all three partners, whether they are male or female, are equal.

This can create a unique dynamic encouraging conditions for growth, development and a lot of fun. The reason for this is simple: In a couple relationship it is very easy for codependent behavior to flourish. This can often take the form of controlling; difficulties in setting clear boundaries; and a host of other problematic behaviors.

It is all too easy for a couple to fall into these unhealthy interaction patterns which, if not dealt with, can often lead to relationship breakdown and

THE TRIAD — MARK, YVONNE AND LISA

failure. When a third person is present — even simply as a witness — many people discover that it's much easier to break out of the cycle of destructive patterns and to choose healthier ways of interacting. When done with love, humor and joy, this process can encourage and stimulate growth, creativity and development. It's no wonder so many artists, writers and other creative and passionate people find this relationship form so rewarding.

Questions you can ask yourself

+ What relationship agreements have my partner and I made with each other? Am I still satisfied with them?
+ What are the different relationships I have? What are the differences between them?
+ What compromises am I prepared to offer in my relationship(s)?
+ How do I let my partner(s) see that I am taking responsibility for my part of the relationship(s)?
+ How do I ensure that I have time for reflection and to make time for myself?
+ What do I think the advantages of a triad could be for me?

Tips for triads

+ Acknowledge the various relationships within the triad. Acknowledge the different dynamic in each relationship and give each relationship sufficient attention.
+ Be open and honest with your partners about your needs. Remember that they do want the best for you, but on the other hand are not always obliged to satisfy your needs.
+ Experience your triad as a journey of discovery. It's not something most have learned how to do and so you will all be learning as you go along.
+ Make clear agreements with each other and reevaluate them regularly. Be prepared to modify agreements if the situation requires it. Both people and circumstances can change over time.
+ Enjoy the double love that you receive. Remember: you are an incredibly lucky person!

Afterword —
Living from Love

*The single most important decision any of us will ever make
is whether or not to believe the universe is friendly.*
— ALBERT EINSTEIN

The ancient Tibetan spiritual and religious discipline of Bon contains a belief that the way we think affects everything we do. Bon beliefs state that understanding and transforming our thoughts is the key to overcoming one of the biggest obstacles in our lives — fear. Many proponents of modern psychology support this view and have taken it further by suggesting that the single most powerful transformational thought we can have is that love, not fear, is the best approach to life. This fits in well with the new solution-oriented (in contrast to the old problem-focused) methods that have been developed over the last years in the realms of both organizational and personal development. These solutions and love-based approaches to life encourage us to see the world as an ongoing joyful, exciting and fun adventure full of opportunities for growth and development. More and more people are choosing to live their lives based on these positive paradigms and are much happier and successful as a result.

As we develop personal lives based on love, more and more of us are discovering that we want to have closer, deeper and more intimate connections with others. Open relationships and polyamory are a part of this awareness. At the same time, many of us who are experiencing this desire also wish to connect with a greater purpose and to be part of creating a better world both for ourselves and for others. So for an increasing number of people there is a direct connection between creating sustainable, authentic and loving intimate relationships and helping to create solutions to the many challenges facing our world. The skills needed to navigate our own personal love lives can indeed be of great use when it comes to loving our world as well.

We hope this book has been informing and inspiring and that it will encourage the development of happy, fulfilling and sustainable relationships for the benefit of us all.

Leonie and Stephan
Amsterdam
March 2010

Acknowledgements —
Stephan

This book has truly been a collective effort inspired by many people, both living and historical. My heartfelt thanks go to:

LEONIE LINSSEN: When I met Leonie for the first time I had the feeling that I knew what it must feel like when, after years of mining, you finally find gold. Her enthusiasm, knowledge, competence, persistence and above all dedication to quality is quite incredible. To top it off she's great fun to work with and has shown remarkable patience during our creative process. The fact that I've found a wonderful new friend as well is truly the icing on the cake.

VICTORIA STAHL: My heartfelt thanks to an amazing woman who, at least in my eyes, must be one of the world's best editors.

The Team at Findhorn Press: THIERRY BOGLIOLO, CAROL SHAW and SABINE WEEKE have been professional, patient and incredibly supportive during a creative process that has taken rather longer than first envisaged. A fantastic publisher indeed!

AUDE FERRIÈRE, DAMIAN KEENAN, RICHARD CROOKES: Much appreciation to Aude for your cheery, bright cover design that graces both the English and Dutch version of the book. Damian must be the most patient designer on the planet – thanks for your persistence! And Richard, your drawings are elegant and concise. Just perfect.

SANDRA, CAROL, FRANZI, VICTORIA, GRIETJE: Many thanks for your copy-editing/proofing assistance.

MARJA DUIN: Ever-cheerful Marja at Archipel provided the crucial input that allowed us to structure the book into a narrative form. I've also discovered that she's quite a talented English-Dutch translator as well as a brilliant editor.

POLY PEOPLE: Polyamory communities, both in-person and virtual, in the US, the UK, the Netherlands, Sweden and Germany have provided me with valuable insights into the lives of real people dealing with real situations. I continue to be amazed at how, given the opportunity, these men and women support and encourage each other in their mutual quest to live richer, congruent and authentic lives.

MONIEK, FRANZI, JOUKO, HILKKA: For clear, honest and unflinching feedback and wonderful friendship.

LAO TZU and all the other Taoists (both mortal and immortal). For their willingness to share insights, explorations and wisdom into the mysterious workings of the Dao.

MIEKE: My beloved partner of 32 years who supports, encourages and gently challenges me. She continually demonstrates what love is.

Stephan Wik
June 2010

Acknowledgements — Leonie

I've been inspired over the years by many people when writing this book. Others have provided rich source material. It is not possible to thank everyone, but there are a few people I'd really like to name:

STEPHAN WIK, my co-author: Thank you for your never-ending enthusiasm and drive, your openness to feedback and your critical and yet supportive manner of questioning. Despite the fact that half-way through our project we decided to start again from scratch, you remained full of hope and were ever cheerful and optimistic. Creating with you was a party – and without you the book would never have happened. I've gained a friend in the process.

MY CLIENTS: I acknowledge you for your openness and trust throughout our many conversations and above all for what I've learned from you. Every person and every relationship is different and I see this again and again. What a privilege it is for me to be invited as a constructive part of your intimate love lives and to see you grow. Thanks to you I have the most enjoyable job in the world, and thanks to you this book has been created.

The hosts, hostesses and guests at Castle Slangenburg: This is the peaceful and in-spiring retreat center where I met Stephan, where the idea for this book was born, and where all the chapters were written. Thanks for your support, our talks and the many questions that were asked, which encouraged clearer explanations.

PETER GERRICKENS: For the creation and publication of your coaching games. The Relationship Game has become an indispensable tool in my work. You've been very supportive of my coaching practice and this book, and I've really enjoyed our wonderful conversations. Thank you for your support and wise advice. In addition, your meaningful feedback on the original text meant deleting and rewriting substan-tial sections. Great!

LOES KOOT, my great colleague: Lots of thanks for your trust in me as a relation-ship coach and for your feedback and tips on the "questions." The book is complete as a result.

LONNEKE ALBERS: Thanks for your lightness of being and your soft and loving approach to life--and for all of the books I was allowed to borrow from you. Your useful feedback allowed me make the background information much clearer for the reader.

MARJA DUIN of Archipel Publishers: Thank you for your thorough editing of the text, your critical questions and observations and the translation of some of the Eng-lish text. It was your idea to create ten "stories" that helped us break the logjam when we were stuck. Ten turned into twelve and you were very enthusiastic as they ap-peared, one after the other. This was a crucial support for us and helped us to trust that we were on the right path.

CHRISTEL, the first woman in my life: A big thank you for your enthusiasm and infectious entrepreneurial spirit and for your belief in me. Our meetings have always been great fun. I'm happy for our friendship!

ADRIETTE EN YVONNE: What incredible women I have as friends! Thanks for all of our special and intimate conversations, and for our friendship. I hope that I can enjoy it long into the future!

MARGA: my ever-cheerful dance and travel partner. Your compassion for the less-fortunate among us is an example for the world. If everyone could have as much love as you do, the world would be a different place.

LION: the most pure and coherent woman I know. Thank you for all the years of friendship we have shared. It's nice to see that time only enhances this – I always feel at home with you.

PETRO, JOKE, MARC, ANJA, KAREL, GE, KARIN, YVONNE, VIVIENNE, ALBERT, LOES EN JEANETTE: my co-trainers and "inter-vision" colleagues. Thanks for the reflections, good questions and tips that I've received from you during our meetings. This has allowed me to know myself better so that I can work better as a relationship coach and an author. Thanks for the laughs!

JACQUELINE LANCÉE: my supervisor. I offer much appreciation for your clear observational ability, your knowledge and your wisdom. I've experienced your unprejudiced view of my speciality as a true gift.

WIES: the most important woman and friend in my life. Your enthusiasm and temperament has given me energy. You are always here for me at the most important times in my life. Thanks for your support and love.

HANS: my childhood love. Thank you for all the things I've learned from you, for your support and for introducing me to Satsang. This has made it clear to me: Everything is Love.

TRUUS EN WIM LINSSEN: my parents. I'm so grateful for your never-ending enthusiasm and for your support. It's so nice to have parents that are supportive and are proud of me especially when what I do is something that is not always accepted in society. I love you.

MIEKE WIK: for your support and softness, the peace you radiate and the space you have given us. Special thanks for your culinary abilities at our meetings which gave Stephan and me the time and space for our creative process.

And last, but not least:

KOOS VAN WEES: my life-parter, my colleague, my everything. Full of trust you let me carry on with this project. It took many weekends when we otherwise would have been together and yet you never once complained. Through you I've been able to experience how important it is to be lovingly accepted--which is the basis of my work. Without your love and support this book would never have happened.

Leonie Linssen
June 2010

Sources of Inspiration
and Further Resources

Love Unlimited web site

The *Love Unlimited* web site can be found at loveunlimited.eu. You can download a sub-set of *The Relationship Game* cards there to use as an exploration tool in your own relationship. There is also an online forum for readers of this book.

Author's web sites

LEONIE'S SITE: www.veranderjewereld.nl
STEPHAN'S SITE: www.wujicentre.com

Useful web sites

LOVING MORE: www.lovemore.com
POLYAMORY FAQ: www.xeromag.com/fvpoly.html
PRACTICAL POLYAMORY: www.practicalpolyamory.com

Polyamory forums

community.livejournal.com/polyamory
forum.polyweekly.com
www.polyamory.com

Coaching games

PETER GERRICKENS, *Het Relatiespel (The Relationship Game)*,
ISBN: 97890 74123 181
PETER GERRICKENS, *Het spel van Verlangen (The Game of Desire)*,
ISBN: 97890-74123-211

Books

CHIA, MANTAK, *The Multi-Orgasmic Couple*, HarperOne, London 2001
COVEY, STEPHEN, *The 7 Habits of Highly Effective People*, Deseret Book Company, New York, NY 2004
JAHNKE, ROGER, *The Healing Promise of Qi*, McGraw-Hill, New York, NY 2002
KINGMA, DAPHNE ROSE, *The Future of Love: The Power of the Soul in Intimate Relationships*, (Doubleday, N.Y. 1999) *http://daphnekingma.com*
KATIE, BYRON, *I Need Your Love - Is That True?*, Three Rivers Press, New York, NY 2006
MCGRAW, DR. PHIL, *Relationship Rescue: Repair Your Relationship Today*, Vermillion, New York, NY 2002
POSTMA, ANNEMARIE, *The Deeper Secret, What does life want from you?*, Watkins, London 2009
ROSENBERG, MARSHALL B., *Nonviolent Communication: a Language of Life*, Puddledancer Press, Encinitas, CA 2003
SMEDES, LEWIS B., *Forgive and Forget: Healing the Hurts We Don't Deserve*, HarperOne, New York, NY 1986
STONE, HAL AND SIDRA, *Embracing Your Inner Critic: Turning Self-Criticism into a Creative Asset*, HarperOne, San Francisco, CA 1993
TEYBER, EDWARD, *Helping Children Cope with Divorce*, Jossey-Bass, Hoboken, NJ 2001
WIK, MIEKE AND STEPHAN, *Beyond Tantra*, Findhorn Press, Findhorn 2005
WILE, DOUGLAS, *The Chinese Sexual Yoga Classics*, State University of New York Press, Albany, NY 1992

FINDHORN PRESS

Life Changing Books

For a complete catalogue,
please contact:

Findhorn Press Ltd
117-121 High Street,
Forres IV36 1AB,
Scotland, UK

t +44 (0)1309 690582
f +44 (0)131 777 2711
e info@findhornpress.com

or consult our catalogue online
(with secure order facility) on
www.findhornpress.com

For information on the Findhorn Foundation:
www.findhorn.org